AORTIC VALVE STENOSIS – CURRENT VIEW ON DIAGNOSTICS AND TREATMENT

Edited by **Petr Šantavý**

Aortic Valve Stenosis – Current View on Diagnostics and Treatment
Edited by Petr Šantavý

Published by InTech
Janeza Trdine 9, 51000 Rijeka, Croatia

Publishing Process Manager Alenka Urbancic

Technical Editor Teodora Smiljanic

Cover Designer InTech Design Team

Additional hard copies can be obtained from orders@intechopen.com

Aortic Valve Stenosis – Current View on Diagnostics and Treatment,
Edited by Petr Šantavý
p. cm.
978-953-307-628-7

For EU product safety concerns:
IN TECH d.o.o., Prolaz Marije Krucifikse Kozulić 3, 51000 Rijeka, Croatia,
info@intechopen.com or visit our website at intechopen.com.

Meet the editor

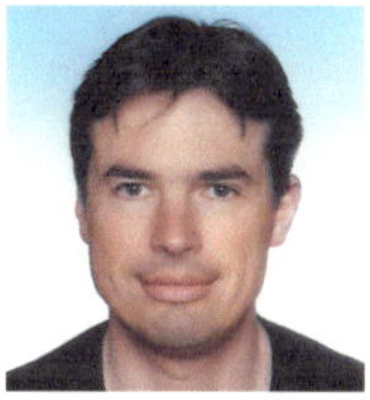

Petr Šantavý graduated from Medical Faculty Palacky University Olomouc, Czech Republic (1998). He received state board exam from general surgery (2001) and specialized in cardiac surgery (2007). He finished his Ph.D. program (2009) based on the work "Aortic bioprosthesis comparison and evaluation of their haemodynamic parameters". He completed a short fellowship at the Jewish Hospital Cardiac Surgery Clinic, Louswille, Kentucky, U.S.A (2007). He worked as a senior registrar at Blackrock Cardiac Surgical Unit in Dublin, Ireland. He is a member of the Czech medical chamber, Ireland medical chamber and European Association of Cardio-Thoracic Surgery. He currently works as a consultant in cardiac surgery at the Dept. of Cardiac Surgery, Palacky Universtity Teaching Hospital, Olomouc, Czech Republic.

Contents

Preface

Aortic stenosis is a major health problem with large personal and economic impact. In the last decades there has been a trend of worldwide aging, and diseases which are common in elderly people will take an important place in clinical practice. Aortic stenosis affects 3-5 percent of persons older than 65 years and leads to greater morbidity and mortality than other cardiac valve diseases. Currently, aortic stenosis is the most frequent heart valve disease in industrialized countries and its prevalence increases with age. Thus with the prolongation of life expectancy, the population of patients with aortic stenosis is expected to grow in the future. The etiology of this disease is changing and is more precisely specified. Diagnostics is changing with new trends and technical developments in echocardiography. Guidelines and indications for aortic valve replacement are changing thanks to new trends in anesthesiology, surgery and mini-invasive approaches. Patients previously considered too old or ill are now indicated for aortic valve replacement procedures.

The approach and management of isolated aortic valve stenosis between fetal life and late adolescence is discussed in the first chapter. Bicuspid aortic valve as a most common form of congenital valve stenosis, is also described. Since approximately 2% of people over the age of 65, 3% of people over the age of 75, and 4% of people over the age of 85 have the disorder, important geriatric aspects of aortic stenosis are discussed in the second chapter. Highly accurate indications are extremely important in future treatment decisions. Abnormal left ventricular response to exercise and change in the hemodynamic severity of the valvular disease add to the prognostic value of clinical symptoms. Therefore stress testing is debated in the third chapter. Successful valve replacement surgery in elderly and often polymorbid patients with congestive heart failure would not be possible without properly aimed modern anesthesia and monitoring. Patients formerly considered inoperable are now profiting from valve replacement procedures. Challenges in anesthesia and post-surgical care are described in chapter four. The only mode of treatment of highly calcified degenerated native aortic valve is its replacement. In chapter five types of surgical approaches and valve prostheses are discussed.

Currently, there is no artificial aortic valve prosthesis hemodynamically equal to native healthy aortic valve. The condition, where the prosthesis orifice is distinctly smaller for a given patient than natively appropriate is defined as patient-prosthesis mismatch. Clinical importance of this phenomenon is the subject of chapter six. Atrial fibrillation is the most common concurrent arrhythmia associated with heart valve diseases and is very poorly tolerated by patients. Sinus rhythm restitution contributes to hemodynamic heart output increase and clinical status improvement. Atrial fibrillation treatment modalities are debated in chapter seven. Despite increasing safeness of standard aortic valve replacement surgery, it is still greatly complex procedure connected with possible adverse complications especially in polymorbid elderly patients. Therefore an effort to decrease extensiveness of surgery has led to development of mini-invasive approaches and procedures. These principles and techniques, which are still evolving, are discussed in the final chapter.

Limited volume of this book cannot substitute comprehensiveness of textbooks, but tries to depict current advances in aortic valve stenosis evaluation and treatment.

Petr Šantavý, M.D., Ph.D.
Dept. of Cardiac Surgery, Palacky Universtity Teaching Hospital, Olomouc,
Czech Republic

1

Congenital Aortic Stenosis in Childhood

David Crespo[1] and Nagib Dahdah[2]
[1]*Hospital Universitario Fundación Alcorcón, Alcorcón, Madrid*
[2]*Sainte-Justine Hospital, Université de Montréal, Montréal, Qc,*
[1]*Spain*
[2]*Canada*

1. Introduction

Aortic valve stenosis is the obstruction to outflow from the left ventricle because of an abnormal aortic valve. The discharge restriction to the systemic ventricle may also be produced by an anomaly at a sub or supravalvar level. Nevertheless, the most common site of occurrence is by far the annulus (70%). Although congenital aortic stenosis is frequently associated with other significant cardiovascular lesions (20%) such as the hypoplastic left heart syndrome, mitral disease and coarctation of the aorta, we will mainly discuss the isolated congenital aortic valve stenosis in this chapter.

Congenital aortic valve stenosis accounts for approximately 5% of all cases of congenital heart disease, with reported incidences ranging from 0.04 to 0.38 per 1000 live births (Botto et al., 2001; Hoffman & Kaplan, 2002). A clear male predominance (Wagner et al., 1977) has been reported, with a gender ratio of 4:1. There is recent evidence of familial predisposition for aortic valve anomalies (recurrence risk ~3% and ~15% in offspring of an affected father or mother respectively). This valvar defect occurs sporadically in most cases however. There is a controversy whether consanguinity has an influence on the incidence of congenital heart disease; while some studies emphasized the increased risk in the rate of congenital cardiac malformations (Badaruddoza et al., 1994; Bassili et al., 2000; Gatrad et al., 1984), others failed to show such association (Robida et al., 1997; Subramanyan et al., 2000). Recent large case series demonstrated that parental consanguinity increases the risk of valvar aortic stenosis as well as atrial septal defect and tetralogy of Fallot, wich supports the involvement of autosomal recessive genes in its bearing (Nabulsi et al., 2003; Chehab et al., 2007). Lately, aortic valvar anomaly in families with autosomal dominant transmission was found to be secondary to a mutation in the *NOTCH1* gene (Garg et al., 2005). This apparent contradiction could be explained by the existence of many cases where a gene may be responsible for autosomal recessive and dominant inheritance, depending on the types of mutations.

Turner syndrome, a congenital disease caused by structural and/or functional aberrations of the X chromosome, is associated with an increased risk of cardiovascular malformations (Bondy & Turner Syndrome Study Group, 2007). It has been reported that 17 to 59% of the patients carrying this chromosomal alteration are affected with at least one structural cardiovascular anomaly, mainly coarctation of the aorta and bicuspid aortic valve, but also mitral valve disease and dilatation of the aortic root (Landin-Wihelmsen et al., 2001; Sybert, 1998). Although some authors have found no correlation between karyotype and heart defects (Poprawski et al., 2009; Ruibal et al., 1997), others reported congenital cardiovascular malformations in 39% of patients with X chromosome monosomy, in 24% with mosaicism and in 12% with structural aberrations (Gravholt, 2001, 2004). The current guideline of the Turner syndrome Study Group (Bondy & Turner Syndrome Study Group, 2007) recommends cardiology assessment including echocardiography. They also recommend physical examination and echocardiography during adolescence and again every 3-5 years in adulthood even if cardiovascular abnormalities were not detected in childhood. Based on the increased risk of hypertension and aortic dissection of these patients, blood pressure should be measured at least twice a year. Girls with bicuspid aortic valve require periodical monitoring for future development of aortic stenosis, regurgitation, and aortic root dilatation.

Bicuspid aortic valve disease is the most common congenital heart defect, with an estimated prevalence of 0.5-2% and male predominance (3:1) (Basso et al., 2004; Roberts, 1970; Ward, 2000). A recent prospective echocardiographic study in newborns showed a high prevalence of 4.6 in 1000 live births (7.1 per 1000 male newborns versus 1.9 per 1000 female newborns) (Tutar et al., 2005). Nowadays, this condition is considered not only a valvar anomaly but a genetic disorder of the aorta and cardiac development (Siu & Silversides, 2010). It is often associated with coarctation of the aorta and dilatation of the thoracic aorta. About 50-75% of patients with coarctation have bicuspid aortic valve (Roos-Hesselink et al., 2003). Other congenital lesions such as ventricular septal defects, patent *ductus arteriosus* or atrial septal defects have been also associated with bicuspid aortic valve. There are few syndromes whose cardiac involvement includes bicuspid aortic valve and left-sided obstructive lesions: Shone syndrome (multiple left-sided anomalies), Williams syndrome (supravalvar stenosis) and Turner syndrome (coarctation of the aorta). The importance of this disease lies in the fact that valvar dysfunction may develop at any time during life span (stenosis or incompetence) as well as disturbances of the aortic wall. In children, 70-85% of stenotic aortic valves are found to be bicuspid (Mack & Silberbach, 2000). An autosomal dominant pattern of inheritance was suggested (Clementi, 1996; McDonald & Maurer, 1989) , and there are reports of 24% prevalence of bicuspid aortic valve in families with more than one affected member (Glick & Roberts, 1994). Recent research demonstrated that bicuspid aortic valve is likely due to mutations in different genes with dissimilar patterns of inheritance (Cripe et al., 2004). The 9% prevalence of bicuspid aortic valve in first-degree relatives of patients with this valvar disturbance supports the current guidelines of the American College of Cardiology/ American Heart Association suggesting echocardiographic screening for bicuspid aortic valve in first-degree relatives (Warnes & American College of Cardiology/ American Heart Association [ACC/AHA], 2008).

2. Anatomical pathology

The obstruction of the left ventricle outflow tract may occur at the subvalvar, valvar or supravalvar levels. Subvalvar stenosis can be produced by a fibrous membrane, a fibromuscular ridge or a diffuse fibromuscular tunnel. Supravalvar obstruction can be a result of an external hourglass deformity with a corresponding luminal narrowing, a fibrous diaphragm or a diffuse narrowing (Edwards, 1965; Iwata et al., 2008). Nevertheles, we will only discuss the most common type at the valvar level, the focus of this chapter. The normal aortic valve is tricuspid, also refered to as trileaflet or trifoliate (3 comissures). The 3 cusps are typically designated as: left coronarian, right coronarian and noncoronarian. Aortic valvar stenosis may be caused by unicuspid, bicuspid or tricuspid valves. Quadricuspid aortic valve is very rare in the exception of the truncus arteriosus malformation.

Unicuspid valve is commonly found in neonates and infants but rare in children, adolescents or adults (Falcone et al., 1971; Mookadam et al., 2010; Roberts & Ko, 2007). All three cusps are fused, with a central opening (acomissural) or an eccentric orifice (unicomissural, with only one fully developed commissure, commonly in a posterior location). It has no attachement or a single lateral attachment to the aorta at the level of the orifice. It is usually observed as a primitive and myxomatous tissue with a pinhole opening, often associated with severe aortic arch obstruction, underdeveloped aortic valve ring, and hypoplastic left heart syndrome. In infants critical stenosis causes a low output syndrome.

Bicuspid (or bileaflet) valve constitutes the most common aortic valve anomaly (Siu & Silversides, 2010). It is clasically formed by 2 unequal-sized leaflets. The larger leaflet has a central raphe resulting from commissural fusion (called "functional" or "fused" bicuspid valve). According to which commissures are fused, there are different morphologic patterns, the most frequent involve fusion of the right and left cusps (60%). Less often, there is no raphe ("pure" or "truly" bicuspid valve). Dilatation of the thoracic aorta is commonly associated with aortic bicuspid valve. It was thought to be secondary to abnormal flow dynamics, but recent evidence indicates structural abnormalities at the cellular level (Niwa et al., 2001; Pachulski et al., 1991). These aberrations are independent of the hemodynamic alteration. They include decreased fibrillin-1, elastin fragmentation and apoptosis. They are thought to play a decisive role in thoracic aorta dilatation and subsequent dissection. These structural anomalies are also found in the main pulmonary artery of patients with bicuspid aortic valves, with unclear clinical significance (De Sa et al., 1999). Obstruction or incompetence of bicuspid aortic valves may develop at any age, mainly in relation to increasing adhesion of remaining commissure margins as well as leaflet thickening or calcification.

Tricuspid valve is the least common cause of congenital aortic stenosis in the youth compared to the various forms of bicuspid valves which represent 70-85% in this age group. The obstruction may be produced by an incomplete leaflet opening and/or cusp thickening, and the stenosis may develop and/or progress over time.

3. Physiopathology

A compensatory left ventricular concentric hypertrophy results proportionally to the degree of the outflow obstruction. A mild stenosis usually produces minimal or no myocardial hypertrophy. The degree of obstruction tends to increase in relation to periods of rapid somatic growth (Wagner et al., 1977). Severe hypertrophy and valvar obstruction may cause myocardial ischemia from the combination of limited cardiac output, reduced coronary perfusion and increased myocardial oxygen consumption. Fibrosis may occur in areas of the myocardium damaged by ischemia (Alsoufi et al., 2007). Post-stenotic aortic root dilatation, defined as dilatation of the vessel wall distal to the area of a partial stenosis, may be caused by the hemodynamic abnormality, but also by intrinsic aortic parietal structural anomalies, especially in bicuspid aortic valve disease. A stenosed aortic valve may also develop valvar incompetence, with secondary left ventricular dilatation in case of significant regurgitation.

During prenatal development, severe aortic stenosis causes increased left cardiac chambers pressures. The blood in the left atrium flows preferencially to the low-pressure right atrium (Alsoufi et al., 2007; Turner et al., 2009). The subsequent reduced antegrade flow through the left heart structures induces detention of left ventricular growth, with the potential development of a hypoplastic left heart syndrome. Occasionally the left ventricle is normal in size, with depressed function of the damaged fibrotic myocardium. The increased afterload contributes to left ventricular hypertrophy and dysfunction. Ventricular hypertrophy and increased intracavitary pressure may lead to subendocardial ischemia with the development of endocardial fibroelastosis which further impairs the ventricular function. In fetuses with aortic stenosis and an intact or restrictive atrial septum, there is no low-pressure outlet for blood entering the left heart, so the left atrium and ventricle may become severely dilated. This may lead to severe mitral regurgitation due to mitral annular dilation, with the resultant elevated pressure and compression of the right heart causing right heart failure, fetal hydrops, and severe pulmonary vascular changes leading to pulmonary hypertension in the neonatal period (Rychik et al., 1999).

4. Clinical manifestations

Although severe stenosis may manifest as exercise induced thoracic pain, fainting, exercise intolerance or even sudden death during childhood, most of the children with valvar aortic stenosis are asymptomatic. The diagnosis is often made during the evaluation of an asymptomatic heart murmur. The typical auscultatory features (Fyler, 1992) consist on an early systolic ejection click followed by a crescendo-decrescendo systolic murmur that reaches peak intensity in mid-systole. In advanced aortic stenosis, the murmur is best heard at the second intercostal space in the right upper sternal border, it radiates to the neck and it is often associated with a systolic thrill in the suprasternal notch. The second sound aortic component is delayed secondary to the left ventricular systole extension, proportionate to the severity of the obstruction. This may result in a narrowly split second heart sound or even with the aortic closure appearing after pulmonary closure (reverse, or paradoxical splitting). The length but not the intensity of the murmur correlates with the degree of the stenosis. The murmur intensity of valvar aortic stenosis increases upon squatting and, in opposition to what happens in cases of hypertrophic obstructive cardiomyopathy, decreases with Valsalva maneuvers. An early diastolic regurgitant murmur may be heard when valvar insufficiency is also present.

Bicuspid aortic valve disease is commonly assymptomatic in childhood; it is estimated that only 1 in 50 children present a clinically significant valve disease by adolescence (Bonow & ACC/AHA, 2008). Globally, only 10-15% of patients present clinical manifestations within the first 12 months of life (Brown et al., 2003; McCrindle et al., 2001). Newborns with critical aortic stenosis usually have a dramatic presentation soon after birth. As the *ductus arteriosus* starts closing, a decreased systemic and coronary perfusion is established. This situation carries a high morbidity and mortality, fatal within hours if left untreated. Neonates and infants with milder stenosis may present with failure to thrive, tachypnea and respiratory distress secondary to pulmonary vascular congestion. Prenatally, only critical stenosis may have clinical repercussion. As previously explained, when an intact or restrictive atrial septum is present, left chambers may become severely dilated leading to heart failure, fetal hydrops and demise. On the other hand, when a non-restrictive *foramen ovale* coexists with critical stenosis, left chambers may be underdeveloped. The myocardium may be damaged, but the systemic output is usually secured at least untill birth through the *ductus arteriosus*.

5. Diagnostic tests

5.1 Electrocardiography

In mild cases there are no electrocardiographic changes. When the stenosis is at least moderate, abnormalities reflecting left ventricular hypertrophy may be observed with or without strain pattern. These findings include increased left ventricular voltages, left bundle-branch block, decreased right anterior forces, T-wave inversion and ST-segment depression. Although electric changes are much more likely with severe stenosis, electrocardiography is not a reliable indicator of the degree of obstruction (Botto et al., 2001; Fowler et al., 1982). In neonates with critical obstruction, the electrocardiogram usually shows right ventricular dominance with evidence of diffuse T-wave and ST-changes secondary to left ventricular strain (Lofland et al., 2001). ACC/AHA guidelines include: "An Electrocardiogram is recommended yearly in the asymptomatic adolescent or young adult with aortic stenosis who has a Doppler mean gradient greater than 30 mmHg or a peak velocity greater than 3.5 m/sec (peak gradient greater than 50 mmHg) and every 2 years if the echocardiographic Doppler mean gradient is less than or equal to 30 mmHg or the peak velocity is less than or equal to 3.5 m/sec (peak gradient less than or equal to 50 mmHg) *(Class I; Level of Evidence C)*" (Bonow & ACC/AHA, 2008).

5.2 Chest X-ray

The heart size is usually normal in children. A prominent ascending aorta is occasionally identifiable because of the dilatation of the ascending aorta, and it is observed as a bulge on the right upper mediastinum or a prominence of the aortic knob on the left upper mediastinum. Those newborns or infants in congestive heart failure due to a critical stenosis show cardiomegaly and pulmonary vascular congestion.

5.3 Echocardiography

Transthoracic echocardiography confirms the diagnosis. The degree of obstruction refers to pressure loss across the valve in systole. This gradient was historically measured by cardiac catheterization. Peak-to-peak gradients determined by cardiac catheterization have constituted the basis of natural history studies and clinical-decision making. Although early investigations suggested that peak Doppler gradient reliably estimated the peak-to-peak catheter gradient (Currie et al., 1985), it was later demonstrated that it consistently overerestimates it by 20-30%, with an exacerbation in presence of significant valvar regurgitation (Baumgartner et al., 1999; Levine et al., 1989; Villavicencio et al., 2003). This is explained by the fact that Doppler technique reflects the maximal instantaneous velocity while peak-to-peak catheter gradient refers to the maximal difference between pressures measured in the left ventricle and the aorta, and also due to the phenomenon of pressure recovery (Clark, 1976). Pressure recovery occurs when the pressure drop across a stenotic orifice is partially recovered distal to the obstruction from conversion of kinetic energy into potential energy. Continuous-wave Doppler measures the point of highest velocity and lowest pressure or vena contracta, so the measured gradients will overestimate the catheter gradient if significant pressure recovery occurs. As higher flow rates secondary to greater resting heart frequencies and small aortas have been shown to exacerbate the phenomenon of pressure recovery (Baumgartner et al., 1999) and both features are often present in children with aortic stenosis. This phenomenon is considered to play an important role while interpreting data derived from ultrasonography studies in this clinical context. To note, pressure recovery has been found to be more significant in mild to moderate aortic valve stenosis (Levine et al., 1989). Moreover, the mean Doppler gradient is a better estimate of the catheter-derived gradients (Fyler, 1992; Levine et al., 1989), although not consistent with the known fluid mechanics principles of left ventricular ejection.

The echocardiogram usually allows to determine with great accuracy the anatomical features of the valve, as well as to identify other cardiovascular lesions which may be associated with this valvulopathy, a subaortic membrane or supravalvar stenosis, if present. A normal aortic valve is formed by three thin cusps which open fully in systole and close completely in diastole. In opposition, a stenotic aortic valve usually has one or two leaflets, usually thick in appearance, with incomplete opening in systole. The parasternal short-axis plane is the best view to identify the number, mobility and thickening of the aortic cusps. A normal aortic valve has a "Y" pattern in diastole and a complete leaflet excursion in systole. It is crucial to explore in detail the hole cardiac cycle, because a bicuspid valve may appear normal in diastole but its typical "fish-mouth" opening can be observed in systole. In addition, the model of systolic opening serves to distinguish a raphe from a commissure. On parasternal long-axis plane (bidimensional and M-mode), a bicuspid valve usually has an eccentric diastolic line of coaptation, whereas a centered line is observed in normal aortic valves. A dome-shaped image secondary to limited excursion of the leaflets is often identified in stenosed aortic valves. The M-mode allows precise measurement of left ventricular function, enlargement and hypertrophy.

The valve area estimate is underused in the typical clinical practice in general. Jet velocity, defined as the antegrade systolic highest velocity across the narrowed aortic valve, is measured using continuous-wave Doppler ultrasound. Accurate data recording mandates multiple acoustic windows in order to determine the peak velocity. Apical and suprasternal or right parasternal most frequently yield the highest velocity. Subcostal or supraclavicular windows are rarely required. Careful patient positioning and adjustment of transducer position and angle are crucial as velocity measurement assumes a parallel intercept angle between the ultrasound beam and direction of blood flow (Baumgartner et al., 2009). Peak Doppler gradient (in mmHg) can be calculated by the modified Bernoulli´s equation: 4 x (jet velocity in m/s)^2. Mean transaortic Doppler pressure gradient is defined as the average difference in pressure between the left ventricle and the aorta during the entire systole. The mean transaortic gradient is easily measured with current echocardiography systems and provides useful information for clinical decision-making. It is calculated by averaging the instantaneous gradients over the ejection period, a function included in most clinical instrument measurement packages using the traced velocity curve. The acoustic windows used to measure the mean Doppler gradient are the same as those used in determining the jet velocity (Baumgartner et al., 2009). Table 1 shows the current classification of the various degrees of aortic stenosis based on the echocardiography.

	Mild stenosis	Moderate stenosis	Severe stenosis
Mean gradient	< 25 mmHg	25-40 mmHg	> 40 mmHg
Jet velocity	< 3 m/s	3-4 m/s	> 4 m/s

Table 1. Aortic stenosis degrees based on echocardiographic parameters in patients without left ventricular dysfunction. Current guidelines of the American College of Cardiology/American Heart Association (ACC/AHA) (Bonow & ACC/AHA, 2008).

A special remark has to be done in reference to ultrasonographic findings of critical aortic stenosis. A small, poorly contracting left ventricle is often observed with varying degrees of endocardial fibroelastosis (seen as areas of increased echogenicity). Hypoplasia of the aortic annulus and the ascending aorta are other commonly associated features. Pulmonary

hypertension may develop secondary to left ventricular failure, causing right ventricular dilatation and tricuspid regurgitation. Finally, the severity of aortic stenosis stratification is not reliable when cardiac function is significantly altered in cases with critical stenosis.
Occasionally associated with aortic stenosis, valvar regurgitation plays a decisive role on clinical decision-making. Although echocardiographic criteria for aortic regurgitation have not been completely established for the pediatric population, some parameters (summarized in Table 2) have been proposed (Snider, 1997; Tribouilloy et al., 1991).

	Mild regurgitation	Moderate regurgitation	Severe regurgitation
Color jet ending	Proximal to the tip of the anterior mitral valve leaflet	Distal to the mitral valve	Distal to the mitral valve
Jet width	< 30%	> 30%	> 30%
Pressure half time	> 600 ms	< 600 ms	< 600 ms
End-diastolic retrograde flow in the descending aorta	< 20 cm/s	20-40 cm/s	> 40 cm/s
Other		Pandiastolic retrograde flow in the abdominal aorta, and dilated left ventricle.	Moderately to severely dilated left ventricle.

Table 2. Aortic regurgitation degrees according to echocardiographic parameters. Jet width refers to the regurgitant flow compared with the left ventricular outflow tract diameter.

ACC/AHA guidelines include: "Doppler echocardiography is recommended yearly in the asymptomatic adolescent or young adult with aortic stenosis who has a Doppler mean gradient greater than 30 mmHg or a peak velocity greater than 3.5 m/sec (peak gradient greater than 50 mmHg) and every 2 years if the Doppler gradient is less than or equal to 30 mmHg or the peak jet velocity is less than or equal to 3.5 m/sec (peak gradient less than or equal to 50 mmHg) *(Class I; Level of Evidence C)"* (Bonow & ACC/AHA, 2008).
Recently, three-dimensional echocardiography became more readily available, permitting "en face" views of intracardiac structures and volumetric measurements (Acar, 2006). In selected patients with valvar aortic stenosis, this emerging imaging technique can be helpful in assessing the morphology and number of leaflets, as well as the degree of fusion between the raphes. It may be useful in the differential diagnosis of valvar and subvalvar obstructions, especially in cases where an infravalvar membrane is very close to the valve and that had not been clearly defined by bidimensional echocardiography (Rubio et al., 2008).
Fetal echocardiography makes a detailed prenatal diagnosis of suspected or known congenital heart disease feasible allowing thus an improved counseling of families; guidance for timing and optimal location of delivery, identification of fetuses requiring specific early postnatal therapy (especially those with ductal dependent lesions such as critical left heart obstructive lesions), and prompt evaluation of genetic syndromes and analysis of the fetal karyotype. It can also serve to identify potential candidates for *in utero* cardiac interventions (Jone & Schowengerdt, 2009). Mild cases of aortic stenosis can be detected prenatally. It is suggested

that prenatal diagnosis of aortic valvar stenosis, and other congenital heart disease alike, is associated with improved postnatal outcome (Chang et al., 1991).

5.4 Cardiac catheterization

The indications of cardiac catheterization for pure diagnostic purposes are very limited nowadays. The catheterization performed at the hemodynamics laboratory with the patient sedated. Peak-to-peak transaortic gradient has been considered for several decades the gold-standard for grading the severity of aortic stenosis. As the aortic systolic pressure is higher and delayed compared to the ventricular pressure (the so-called "standing wave effect") (Lock, 1987), it is not recommended to compare pressures between left ventricle and a distal artery (such as a femoral artery) in order to avoid a gradient underestimation. Other parameters including degree of aortic regurgitation, cardiac output, left ventricular systolic function and aortic annulus diameter can be also determined during catheterization.

Diagnostic cardiac catheterization is currently recommended for adolescents and young adults, equally valid for children, in the following situations (Bonow & ACC/AHA, 2008):

Cardiac catheterization for the evaluation of aortic stenosis is an effective diagnostic tool in the asymptomatic adolescent or young adult when results of Doppler echocardiography are equivocal regarding severity of aortic stenosis or when there is a discrepancy between clinical and noninvasive findings regarding severity of aortic stenosis *(Class I; Level of Evidence C).*

Cardiac catheterization is indicated in the adolescent or young adult with aortic stenosis who has symptoms of angina, syncope, or dyspnea on exertion if the Doppler mean gradient is greater than 30 mmHg or the peak velocity is greater than 3.5 m/sec (peak gradient greater than 50 mmHg) *(Class I; Level of Evidence C).*

Cardiac catheterization is indicated in the asymptomatic adolescent or young adult with aortic stenosis who develops T-wave inversion at rest over the left precordium if the Doppler mean gradient is greater than 30 mmHg or the peak velocity is greater than 3,5 m/sec (peak gradient greater than 50 mmHg) *(Class I; Level of Evidence C).*

Cardiac catheterization for the evaluation of aortic stenosis is a reasonable diagnostic tool in the asymptomatic adolescent or young adult who has a Doppler mean gradient greater than 40 mmHg or a peak velocity greater than 4 m/sec (peak gradient greater than 64 mmHg) *(Class IIa; Level of Evidence C).*

Cardiac catheterization for the evaluation of aortic stenosis is reasonable in the adolescent or young adult who has a Doppler mean gradient greater than 30 mmHg or a peak velocity greater than 3.5 m/sec (peak gradient greater than 50 mmHg) if the patient is interested in athletic participation or becoming pregnant, or if the clinical findings and the Doppler echocardiographic findings are disparate *(Class IIa; Level of Evidence C).*

5.5 Exercise testing

Exercise testing can be useful in borderline cases (e.g., in patients interested in engaging in vigorous physical activities), but should be avoided in symptomatic patients owing to a high risk of complications. Stress testing can identify a limited exercise capacity, abnormal blood pressure responses, exercise-induced symptoms or electrocardiographic changes (ST-segment depression or T-wave inversion). A significant obstruction may be present when any of these abnormalities is identified. ACC/AHA guidelines refer to exercise testing as follows: "Graded exercise testing is a reasonable diagnostic evaluation in the adolescent or young adult with aortic stenosis who has a Doppler mean gradient greater than 30 mmHg or a peak velocity greater than 3.5 m/sec (peak gradient greater than 50 mmHg) if the patient is interested in athletic participation, or if the clinical findings and Doppler findings are disparate *(Class IIa; Level of Evidence C)*" (Bonow & ACC/AHA, 2008).

5.6 Holter monitor

The prevalence of serious ventricular arrhythmias (multiform premature ventricular contractions, ventricular couplets and ventricular tachycardia) is increased in patients with aortic stenosis. When the invasive peak-to-peak gradient is over 50 mmHg there is a higher incidence of sudden death (Keane et al., 1993; Wolfe et al., 1993). Considering that a clear consensus is well stated for the clinical decision-making of mild and severe cases (medical follow-up and intervention, respectively), Holter monitoring may be a useful tool in those patients with a moderate degree of aortic stenosis, but evidence based data is unavailable.

5.7 Magnetic resonance

Cardiovascular magnetic resonance has emerged as an alternative noninvasive imaging without ionizing radiation, particularly useful in patients with poor acoustic windows. It provides precise images of valve anatomy and allows quantitative evaluation of stenosis and regurgitation (Cawley at al., 2009). Delayed myocardial enhancement magnetic resonance can serve to delineate the location and transmural extent of endocardial fibroelastosis in infants, thus providing an accurate roadmap for the surgical planning of fibroelastosis resection and for monitoring the results (Tworetzky et al., 2005). Magnetic resonance is also proposed to aid fetal ultrasonography in the prenatal assessment of congenital cardiac malformations (Manganaro et al., 2008).

6. Natural course

Critical aortic stenosis produces severe congestive heart failure and shock in fetuses, neonates and infants. It usually leads to death within hours or days if left untreated. Before the era of surgery, it was estimated that aortic valvar stenosis presenting within the first year of life carried a mortality rate of 23% (Campbell, 1968). In a necropsy series of 26 children with aortic stenosis under 15 years old, 43% died within the first month of life and 77% within the first year (Samánek et al., 1988). Beyond these ages, children with untreated severe aortic stenosis seldom live more than 5 years from the time of diagnosis, similar to life expectancy reported in adults (Kitchiner et al., 1993; Wagner et al., 1977). The survival of patients with mild obstruction is slightly lower than that of the general population, probably related to sporadic deceases secondary to infective endocarditis or to unexpected quick incremental severity (Keane et al., 1993; Kitchiner et al., 1993). In patients with moderate obstruction who receive no treatment, the reported survival rate is 72.2% at 5 years and 45.6% at 20 years (Kitchiner et al., 1993).

The report from the Natural History Study of Congenital Heart Defects which included 462 patients with aortic stenosis (60% between 2-11 years and 24% between 11-21 years at initial evaluation), observed that the obstruction tends to increase over time, especially in cases with higher gradients on enrolment. Whereas only 20% of those patients with initial peak-

to-peak transaortic gradient lower than 25 mmHg at initial catheterization required a cardiac intervention during 25 years of follow-up, children with baseline peak-to-peak transaortic gradient over 50 mmHg were at risk for serious cardiovascular events, including arrhythmias, endocarditis and sudden death, at a rate of 1.2% per year (Keane et al., 1993; Kitchiner et al., 1993). The rate of aortic stenosis progression is highly variable and appears to be age related. It is fast in infants, moderate in children and slow in adolescents; probably related to the inability of the valve orifice to increase in proportion to somatic growth (el-Said et al., 1972). In line with this assumption, a study in which 129 children with aortic stenosis were followed periodically with serial echocardiograms, showed that 89% of children under 2 years old and 61% of children over 2 years old experimented progression of the obstruction (Kiraly et al., 2003). Although significant and progressive aortic regurgitation is commonly acquired after surgery or percutaneous balloon valvuloplasty, it can also occur in patients with untreated aortic stenosis (Keane et al., 1993).
Sudden death, with an average incidence of 0.3% per year (Keane et al., 1993), occurs almost exclusively in patients with a peak Doppler gradient higher than 50 mmHg even in the absence of symptoms (Keane et al., 1993; Otto et al., 1997). About half of these fatal events occur during or immediately after exercise (Lambert et al., 1974). Bacterial endocarditis occurs in 1-4% of patients with untreated aortic stenosis (18-31 per 10000 patient-years) (Campbell, 1968; Gersony et al., 1993; Hossack et al., 1980). The risk is present in mild cases, with higher incidence in patients with more severe stenosis. Aortic regurgitation does not seem to increase the risk of developing bacterial endocarditis however (Gersony et al., 1993).
Clinical presentation of patients with bicuspid aortic valve varies from severe valve disease in infancy to asymptomatic valve or thoracic aorta disease in the older child, but symptoms usually develop in adulthood (Siu & Silversides, 2010). Although aortic stenosis can be present in children secondarily to a small valve orifice, the valve usually has none or mild degree of obstruction in childhood and experience a progressive worsening over time because of sclerosis and calcification (Chui et al., 2001). High levels of serum cholesterol have been associated with an acceleration of the sclerosing process of the bicuspid valve (Chui et al., 2001). A study performed on adult patients with bicuspid aortic valves showed a median increase of 0.7 mmHg per year in peak Doppler gradient (Tzemos et al., 2008). Pure aortic incompetence due to a prolapsed leaflet may occur in childhood but is more likely to develop and progress later in time; nevertheless, this remains an infrequent cause of intervention requirement even in adults. Aortic root dilatation has been documented in childhood, suggesting that this process begins early in life (Beroukhim et al., 2006; Gurvitz et al., 2004). Its progression is more likely in children with a larger aorta at baseline, but it is extremely rare to necessitate intervention before adulthood (Holmes et al., 2007).

7. Management

Balloon aortic valvoplasty constitutes the therapeutic procedure of choice in most centers for the treatment of congenital aortic stenosis (Khalid et al., 2006). Other interventional options, including both surgical and hybrid techniques and also fetal intervention are also discussed.

7.1 Balloon aortic valvoplasty

Balloon aortic valvoplasty, first described in the early 1980s, is a widely used technique in the treatment of valvar aortic stenosis in children (Lababidi, 1983; Lababidi et al., 1984). The technique is performed under deep sedation, with the exception of the neonates and the critically ill patients. Vascular access is usually obtained with a retrograde approach using the femoral artery. In neonates and small infants, other sites of access have been used in order to avoid the risk of femoral arterial compromise (Weber, 2006). These include:

The umbilical artery route was initially advocated as a way to avoid femoral artery injury in view of the large diameter balloon dilatation catheters that were available at the time (Beekman et al., 1991). Although technically feasible, it may be difficult to traverse the tortuous umbilical-iliac artery system, may introduce bacteria from the umbilicus and may cause excessive loss of blood during wire and catheter exchanges.

The right scapular artery was reported to be safe and effective in infants with critical aortic valve stenosis (Alekyan et al., 1995). It typically requires surgical exposure of the artery and is contraindicated in the presence of an aberrant right subclavian artery.

The anterograde transvenous approach may be performed via the *foramen ovale* or by a transeptal puncture when the atrial septum is intact (Hausdorf et al., 1993). This procedure spares the femoral arteries for potential future use but may be technically challenging and may cause mitral valve damage.

The right carotid artery was firstly used based on the extensive experience with carotid artery cannulation for extracorporeal membrane oxigenation in newborns (Fischer et al., 1990). it is reported to be effective and safe, and it allows performing the entire procedure at the bedside with the aid of continuous transesophageal echocardiographic guidance, thus avoiding the use of fluoroscopy (Weber et al., 2000). Its disadvantages include the risk of carotid artery injury with potential neurologic complications and the need of surgical exposure.

Above all, the retrograde femoral arterial approach remains the most commonly used. The potential associated complications have been significantly reduced with the availability of low profile diameter balloons. Once the vascular access is assured, the aortic annulus diameter and the degree of aortic regurgitation are determined, a complete right and left cardiac catheterization is performed and the peak-to-peak transaortic gradient is determined from simultaneous or sequential measurements of left ventricular and ascending aorta pressures.

Balloon aortic valvoplasty is contraindicated when an aortic regurgitation of moderate or higher degree is present, and it is not recommended if the valve is significantly calcified. It is performed in cases of critical aortic stenosis with variable institutional preferences. Recommendations for aortic balloon valvoplasty in adolescents and young adults, which may be applied to children, are the following (Bonow & ACC/AHA, 2008):

Aortic balloon valvotomy is indicated in the adolescent or young adult patient with aortic stenosis who has symptoms of angina, syncope, or dyspnea on exertion and a catheterization peak LV-to-peak aortic gradient greater than or equal to 50 mmHg without a heavily calcified valve *(Class I; Level of Evidence C).*

Aortic balloon valvotomy is indicated for the asymptomatic adolescent or young adult patient with aortic stenosis who has a catheterization peak LV-to-peak aortic gradient greater than 60 mmHg *(Class I; Level of Evidence C).*

Aortic balloon valvotomy is indicated in the asymptomatic adolescent or young adult patient with aortic stenosis who develops ST or T-wave changes over the left precordium on ECG at rest or with exercise and who has a catheterization peak LV-to-aortic gradient greater than 50 mmHg *(Class I; Level of Evidence C).*

Aortic balloon valvotomy is reasonable in the asymptomatic adolescent or young adult patient with aortic stenosis when catheterization peak LV-to-peak aortic gradient is greater than 50 mmHg and the patient wants to play competitive sports or desires to become pregnant *(Class IIa; Level of Evidence C).*

In the adolescent or young adult patient with aortic stenosis, aortic balloon valvotomy is probably recommended over valve surgery when balloon valvotomy is possible. Patients should be referred to a center with expertise in balloon valvotomy *(Class IIa; Level of Evidence C).*

Aortic balloon valvotomy should not be performed when the asymptomatic adolescent or young adult patient with aortic stenosis has a catheterization peak LV-to-peak aortic gradient less than 40 mmHg without symptoms or ECG changes *(Class III; Level of Evidence C).*

The recommended size of the balloon for the valvoplasty is 80-90% of the measured aortic annulus; smaller ones may not be able to accurately relief the obstruction. If the reduction in gradient is below 50% or the residual gradient is higher than 50 mmHg and the degree of insufficiency remains less than moderate, sequential progressive dilatations using larger balloons may be performed, but the size of the balloon may not exceed 120% of the diameter of the valvar ring in order to avoid iatrogenic regurgitation (McCrindle et al., 1996; Phillips et al., 1987; Sholler et al., 1988). The balloon is carefully positioned across the aortic valve and then inflated until the waist produced by the valve on the balloon disappears. This technique can be performed by using one balloon, or two for large diameter valves. In the double-balloon valvoplasty, two separate arterial catheters are used to cross the aortic valve. The typical flattening of the balloons against each other during inflation mandates a higher ratio of the sum of the balloons nominal diameters to valve annulus to around 130% (both with similar diameter and length); the two balloons are positioned across the valve and inflated simultaneously. The results in terms of gradient relief and degree of iatrogenic aortic regurgitation are similar when compared to the single-balloon procedure, with the additional advantages to reduce vessel trauma and to avoid the complete obstruction of the left ventricular outflow tract as would occur during inflation of a single large balloon (Beekman et al., 1988; Mullins et al., 1987). The rapid movements of the inflated balloon up and down at the left ventricular outflow tract during valvoplasty, is thought to favor aortic insufficiency (Daehnert et al., 2004). Hence, different maneuvers such as the use of more rigid wires, induced asystole with adenosine or ventricular fibrillation have been employed aiming to improve balloon stability (Kahn et al., 1998, 2000). Rapid ventricular pacing, is an alternative effective and safe way to stabilize the balloon. It consists on electrically stimulating the right ventricle rapidly to accelerate the ventricular frequency until a 50% systolic aortic pressure drop is achieved, and inflating the balloon at this point (David et al., 2007). An effective relief of the obstruction is usually achieved by the valvoplasty, with a 50-70% reduction of the pressure gradient in children with isolated aortic stenosis and in those with associated cardiovascular lesions (Crespo et al., 2009; Gatzoulis et al., 1995; Kusa et al., 2004; McCrindle et al., 1996; Rao et al., 1989). Independent risk factors for suboptimal gradient reduction are high pre-valvoplasty transaortic gradient, children aged less than a month or more than 14 years, high pre-procedural left ventricle end diastolic pressure, the use of a balloon to annulus ratio less than 0.9, and fused bicuspid valve as opposed to pure bicuspid valve (Crespo et al., 2009; Kusa et al., 2004; McCrindle et al., 1996). Repeated balloon dilatation, and valvoplasty for residual stenosis after surgical valvotomy seem to be efficient (Crespo et al., 2009; Meliones et al., 1989; Phillips et al., 1987; Shim et al., 1997; Sholler et al., 1988). Valvoplasty may cause aortic regurgitation as the result of commissural avulsion, cusp dehiscence and or tear perforation. This iatrogenic regurgitation, which was described to be associated with fused bicuspid valves (Reich et al., 2004), has been proven to be related to oversized balloons which lead to improve practice and guidelines, therefore high degrees of immediate post procedural insufficiency became uncommon (McCrindle et al., 1996; Phillips et al., 1987; Sholler et al., 1988). The rate of at least moderate aortic regurgitation shortly after the procedure is between 7.3-22.6% and may progress afterwards (Crespo et al., 2009; Fratz et al., 2008; McCrindle et al., 1996; McElhinney et al., 2005; Reich et al., 2004). Iatrogenic aortic insufficiency, severe hypotension, ventricular arrhythmias, vessel damage, complete atrioventricular block, cardiac tamponade and mitral valve injury are the main serious procedural related complications. In a large multi-institutional series of 630 balloon dilatations which did not exclude children with associated cardiovascular anomalies major complications occured in 7.1%, significantly more frequent in newborns (McCrindle et al., 1996). Mortality attributable to the valvoplasty varies between 0 and 2.1%, again with a clearly higher incidence during the neonatal period (Kusa et al., 2004; McCrindle et al., 1996; Crespo et al., 2009; Moore et al., 1996). Both progressive worsening of aortic regurgitation and an increase in residual transvalvar gradient seem to be inevitable. Aortic inssuficiency of at least moderate grade varies between 22.3% and 35% after 5 to 5.3 years (McElhinney et al., 2005; Reich et al., 2004) and is about 50% at 7.5 years follow-up interval (Pedra et al., 2003). The increase in residual transvalvar gradient, or restenosis, varies between 0% and 32.1% according to different definitions of residual gradients used by different investigators (Balmer et al., 2004; Rao et al., 1989; Reich et al., 2004). In a very recent series, including both neonates and older children, 10% of the patients needed reintervention in the long term due to restenosis (Fratz et al., 2008). The survival rate after valvoplasty at 6 and 14.4 years varies between 93% and 100% in older children (Fratz et al., 2008; Galal et al., 1997; Moore et al., 1996; Reich et al., 2004), whereas it varies between 71–74.6% (Fratz et al., 2008; McElhinney et al., 2005) and 71% (Reich et al., 2004) at 10 and 14.4 years respectively when performed in the neonatal period. The freedom from reintervention at mid and long-term follow up varies between 46 and 76% (Fratz et al., 2008; Galal et al., 1997; Moore et al., 1996; Rao, 1999; Reich et al., 2004) after 8–14.4 years in older children, whereas it varies between 47–57.6% (Fratz et al., 2008; McElhinney et al., 2005; Villalba et al., 2002) and 26% (Reich et al., 2004) at 5–10 years and 14.4 years respectively when performed in the neonatal period. A significant decrease in dispersion of the ventricular repolarisation is reported following valvoplasty in patients with severe congenital aortic stenosis, which would theoretically diminish the electrical instability, preventing ventricular arrhythmias later on in life (Sarubbi et al., 2004). In conclusion, balloon valvoplasty is a safe an effective method for the treatment of congenital aortic valve stenosis, constituting the therapeutic procedure of choice in most centers.

7.2 Fetal intervention

Congenital heart disease constitutes the most frequent congenital anomaly and the main cause of death among infants in the United States, thus it is an attractive target for prenatal diagnosis and therapy (Turner et al., 2009). In the case of critical aortic stenosis, early *in utero* relief of the obstruction is thought to reverse the progression toward left ventricular hypoplasia (De Oliveira et al., 2004; Tweddell et al., 2002). As hypoplastic left heart syndrome is one of the most severe congenital heart defects that requires multi-staged palliative surgery or even heart transplantation, severe aortic valve stenosis is the defect for which fetal intervention is most likely to be considered (Brown et al., 2003; McCrindle et al., 2001; McElhinney et al., 2005). The aim of fetal aortic valvuloplasty is to relief the left obstruction of the ventricle outlet to prevent progression to endocardial fibroelastosis and ventricle hypoplasia. Some echocardiographic features found in midgestation fetuses with aortic stenosis and normal left ventricle length including retrograde flow in the transverse arch, left-to-right flow across the *foramen ovale,* monophasic mitral inflow and left ventricular dysfunction have been reported to predict progression to hypoplastic left heart syndrome (Makikallio et al., 2006). Fetal aortic valvuloplasty must be performed in the early second trimester. The procedure can be performed by laparotomy to expose the uterus or by uterine incision and fetal exposure. These invasive techniques offer better ultrasound imaging quality and shorter distance to the fetal heart, but they carry the risk of increased maternal morbidity and premature delivery. For these reasons less invasive techniques are preferred. Under bidimensional ultrasound guidance, a 19G cannula and stylet needle are advanced through the maternal abdomen, uterine wall and fetal chest wall, accessing the fetal heart by the left ventricle. The valvoplasty is performed with a small coronary artery balloon over a thin, floppy guide wire. The balloon is inflated and the procedure is considered successful if there is clear evidence of increased anterograde flow across the valve and/or new aortic regurgitation by color-Doppler (Marshall et al., 2005; McElhinney et al., 2009; Wilkins-Haug et al., 2006). Complications of valvoplasty in the fetus include bradycardia (50% upon needle access to the ventricle), pericardial effusion, significant iatrogenic aortic regurgitation and fetal demise. Boston Children´s Hospital has the largest experience with the technique (McElhinney et al., 2009): 70 interventions were attempted in fetuses expected to progress to hypoplastic left heart syndrome without intervention; 52 procedures were considered successful (74%); hemodynamic changes (bradycardia and ventricular dysfunction) treated with intramuscular and/or intracardiac medications and/or hemopericardium for which drainage was attempted occurred in 28 fetuses (40%) (Mizrahi-Arnaud et al., 2007); moderate or severe aortic regurgitation was noted in 20 fetuses (38%), resolved or improved to mild regurgitation in all but 1 case. In the Boston series, 1 pregnancy was terminated and 8 others (13% total) ended in fetal death or preterm stillbirth. The rate of growth of the left cardiac structures was greater among fetuses that underwent successful intervention. Finally, 20 of the 70 patients (29%) achieved the ultimate goal of biventricular circulation.

In conclusion, fetal aortic valvoplasty may be useful in fetuses with aortic stenosis. The potential benefits of the procedure must be weighted against the inherent serious risks. Based on the current knowledge, fetal aortic valvoplasty should not be performed in fetuses with aortic stenosis that will not otherwise progress to hypoplastic left heart syndrome.

7.3 Surgery

Two opposed clinical situations have to be considered when referring to surgical procedures in aortic stenosis. The single-ventricle end of the spectrum is characterized by a severe degree of underdevelopment of the left heart-aorta complex, resulting in obstruction to the systemic cardiac output and the inability of the left heart to support the systemic circulation. The two-ventricle end of the spectrum is characterized by a normal or moderately underdeveloped left heart-aorta complex, able to fully support the systemic circulation.

7.3.1 Two-ventricle repair

Surgical valvotomy is of historic interest and is rarely used as first attempt in children. When balloon aortic valvoplasty is ineffective or significant aortic regurgitation is present, valve repair or replacement may be necessary (Bonow & ACC/AHA, 2008).

7.3.1.1 Valvotomy

Open valvotomy with cardiopulmonary bypass, firstly described in 1958 (Spencer et al., 1958), has remained the main therapeutic option for congenital aortic stenosis in neonates and infants until the advent of balloon valvoplasty in the early 1980s. It offers the advantage of a detailed examination of the valve and accurate valvotomy, in opposition to the blind dilatation of the balloon procedure. Its main disadvantages are the morbidity and mortality related to the surgery and the cardiopulmonary bypass, and an increase in the complexity of a future surgery due to redo sternotomy. The operation is performed on cardiopulmonary bypass with mild hypotermia, through median sternotomy (Hraska et al., 2007). The anterior part of the aortic root is dissected to identify the origin of the right coronary artery, and the aorta is incised 5-10 mm above the origin of the coronary artery. Holding sutures are placed on the edges of the aortotomy and the aortic valve is carefully examined. Finally, the fused commissures are carefully divided, ensuring that the leaflets are well supported and not liable to prolapse. Other techniques such as closed transventricular valvotomy have been also used for the initial management of critical neonatal aortic stenosis in some centers (Brown et al., 2006). Both the reduction of the transaortic gradient (53-67%) and the creation of significant aortic regurgitation (8-21%) after the surgical valvotomy are similar to those described for the valvoplasty technique (Alexiou et al., 2001; Brown et al., 2003; Miyamoto et al., 2006; Zafra et al., 1993). Early mortality after neonatal surgical aortic valvotomy was very high in the early experience but was significantly reduced in subsequent publications, with rates varying between 2.1% and 18% (Alexiou et al., 2001; Bhabra et al., 2003; Brown et al., 2003; Gildein et al., 1996; Hawkins et al., 1998; Miyamoto et al., 2006; Zain et al., 2006). Several risk factors for increased operative mortality include endocardial fibroelastosis, hypoplastic left ventricle, hypoplastic aortic annulus, associated cardiovascular anomalies, extremely small neonates, earlier era surgery, monocuspid aortic valve and impaired left ventricular function (Bhabra et al., 2003; Brown et al., 2006; Hawkins et al., 1998; Miyamoto et al., 2006). Similarly to what happens after balloon dilatation, progressive worsening of aortic insufficiency and re-stenosis occurs at long-term follow up after surgical valvotomy. The freedom from reintervention is 80-85% after 5-7 years (Brown et al., 2006; Cobanoglu & Dobbs, 1996; Miyamoto et al., 2006), 55-78% after 10 years (Alexiou et al., 2001; Brown et al., 2006; Hawkins et al., 1998; Miyamoto et al., 2006) and 53-65% after 15-20 years (Brown et al., 2006; Miyamoto et al., 2006). Long-term survival rate is 74-100% at 5-10 years (Alexiou et al., 2001; Bhabra et al., 2003; Brown et al., 2003; Cowley et al., 2001; Gaynor et al., 1995; Hawkins et al., 1998) and 84-88% at 15-20 years (Brown et al., 2003; Gaynor et al., 1995). A retrospective review of infants undergoing primary surgical aortic valvotomy showed better long-term outcomes (in terms of survival and freedom from reintervention) when surgery resulted in trileaflet rather than bileaflet anatomy (Bhabra et al., 2003).

7.3.1.2 Repair procedures

When the aortic stenosis coexists with a severe degree of valvar incompetence both primarily or after a first approach by either balloon dilatation or surgical valvotomy, some authors have proposed reconstructive techniques such as reattachment of an avulsed cusp to the aortic annulus, relief of commissural fusion and debridement of thickened cusps instead of valvar replacement (Alsoufi et al. 2006; Bacha et al., 2001; Hawkins et al., 1996; Odim et al., 2005; Polimenakos et al., 2010; Schäfers et al.; 2008). Bicuspidisation procedure, whose principles are elevation of the comissure and augmentation of the cusps, has been advocated for unicuspid aortic valves (Schäfers et al.; 2008). This conversion into bicuspid anatomy has been reported to have no mortality, good functional results and appropriate freedom from reintervention (67%) and from valve replacement (100%) at 4 years. Other non replacement strategy is aortic cusp extension valvuloplasty with selective use of tricuspidization (Polimenakos et al., 2010). Pericardial cusp extension counteracts the valve's inherent sinuses of Valsalva shallowness, reestablishes normal depth of the sinuses, secures adequate and longer coaptation surface and restores the normal "crownlike" appearance of the valve; while tricuspidization ensures a larger central opening and minimizes turbulence. This technique has been proven to effectively reduce aortic insufficiency and regurgitation, and to improve left ventricular wall thickness and dimensions in infants and children. Its long-term outcomes at 1, 5 and 10 years are 97, 71 and 51% free from moderate or greater aortic regurgitation; 97, 67 and 54% free from moderate or greater aortic stenosis; and 97, 71 and 56% free from aortic valve replacement.

7.3.1.3 Aortic valve replacement

7.3.1.3.1 Ross operation

The Ross operation was firstly described in 1967 (Ross, 1967). It was initially considered too complex by the surgical community and was relegated to single curiosity until 1988, when its long-term results were reported (Ross, 1988). The Ross procedure consists on aortic valve replacement with a pulmonary autograft. During the operation, the pulmonary native valve was substituted by a homograft in the first series, or alternatively by a valved conduit in subsequent practice constituted by a gluterhaldeheyde preserved bovine jugular vein. When the left ventricular outflow tract is enlarged during the procedure, then the surgery is denominated Ross-Konno (Reddy et al., 1996). The Ross operation appeared to be the panacea of aortic valve replacements for growing infants and children due to the excellent hemodynamic performance and growing capacity of the autograft, the long-term expected durability of the homograft and a very low thrombogenecity which makes anticoagulant therapy unnecessary (Elkins, 1999; Oury, 1996), but some patients did require reoperations because of autograft or homograft failure and progressive dilatation of the neo-aortic root. New improvements were applied to prevent neoaortic root dilatation and autograft regurgitation using graft inclusion techniques. A Ross operation may be considered whenever replacement of the aortic valve is indicated, especially in the youngest patients. Moreover, it is contraindicated in case of primary or iatrogenic lesions of the pulmonary valve for obvious reasons, in Marfan syndrome and in autoimmune tissue diseases (Corno et al., 2001). Early mortality is 1-2.5% (Brown et al., 2009; Kouchoukos et al., 2004; Oury et al., 1998) with a 10-15-year survival rate of 96-98% (Brown et al., 2009; Kouchoukos et al., 2004), observing significantly better outcomes for children older than 1 year of age compared to children under 1 year (Brown et al., 2009). In a large series with infants, children and adults, overall freedom from reoperation was 91% at 15 years (Brown et al., 2009). In a study on older children and young adults, event-free survival (freedom from death, reoperation, thromboembolism and endocarditis) was 93% at 5 years, 78% at 7 years, and 73% at 10 years postoperatively (Kouchoukos et al., 2004). A recent series of 27 infants less than 18 months of age who underwent the Ross procedure showed 3 early and no late deaths, and freedom for reintervention of 87% at 8 years (Williams et al., 2005).

7.3.1.3.2 Mechanical valve replacement

The selection of the most appropriate substitute in children with irreparable aortic valve lesion remains controversial. The first mechanical model was the caged-ball mechanical prosthesis, used in the 1960s and early 1970s. The xenograft valve was introduced in the early to mid-1970s and was initially considered better suited for children, but unfortunately these valves demonstrated early failure (Robbins et al., 1988). The new generation mechanical valves exhibit minimal structural degeneration, but continue to be prone to valve-related complications. Mechanical prosthetic valves carry the risks of thromboembolism, requiring anticoagulation. The use of these valves also faces the need of iterative replacement because of the valve outgrowth in the growing young patient. Nevertheless, its safety and reproducible implantation technique, good hemodynamic performance, low incidence of valve-related events, acceptable short and long-term outcomes and prolonged durability, convert it into a good alternative in cases where aortic valve replacement is mandatory (Alexiou et al., 2000). The longevity of mechanical prostheses is superior compared to bioprosthetic valves, but its implantation has been associated with very high early re-intervention rate and poor survival in neonates and small infants, limiting its use in these ages (Karamlou et al., 2005). Aortic valve replacement using mechanical prosthetic valves in children often requires annular enlargement to insert commercially available prostheses. This enlargement can be performed by different techniques: the Konno procedure involves incision of the ventricular septum, which might cause ventricular dysfunction, atrioventricular conduction block or arrhythmias; the Manouguian procedure with extension of the incision to the anterior mitral leaflet might cause mitral inssufficiency; and Yamaguchi procedure with an anterior incision in the aortic annulus is directed into the commissure between the right and left coronary cusps continued downward across the aortic ring to near full thickness of the right ventricular wall, is nowadays the technique of choice because it does not damage the ventricular septum or the mitral valve (Masuda et al., 2008). Operative death rate varies between 0-5% in several series (Alexiou et al., 2000; Karamlou et al., 2005; Masuda et al., 2008; Mazzitelli et al., 1998; Popov et al., 2009; Turrentine et al., 2001), mostly involving children with severe preoperative pulmonary hypertension or myocardial dysfunction. Although previous series showed worse outcomes, more recent studies report actuarial survival of 89-95% at 10 years (Alexiou et al., 2000; Turrentine et al., 2001), 87-92% at 15 years (Masuda et al., 2008) and 85% at 20 years (Alexiou et al., 2000). Freedom from surgical re-intervention ranges between 80-92% at 10 years (Alexiou et al., 2000; Champsaur et al., 1997; Mazzitelli et al., 1998; Turrentine et al., 2001), 85-86% at 15 years (Alexiou et al., 2000; Turrentine et al., 2001) and 54-86% at 20 years (Alexiou et al., 2000; Mazzitelli et al., 1998). A very recent series from Japan of 45 children with a median follow-up of 9.2 years showed excellent outcomes, with an actuarial freedom from reoperation of 94% at 15 years (Masuda et al., 2008). This publication also noted that 40 of the 42 (95%) survivors had a peak Doppler gradient less than 3 m/s at the latest evaluation. This finding endorses the previous report of 44 of the 50 (88%) survivors being in NYHA class I with a mean Doppler gradient across the aortic prosthesis of 17.9 mmHg at last follow-up (mean follow-up of 7.7 years) (Alexiou et al., 2000), thus highlighting the importance of the functional status and the hemodynamic performance. Some authors have observed a correlation among transprosthetic flow velocity and manufactured valve area, suggesting that implantation of mechanical valves of 19 mm or larger may not require further re-replacement (Masuda et al., 2008; Shanmugan et al., 2005). This is obviously a clear limitation for the low spectrum of the pediatric age group.

7.3.2 Single-ventricle repair

The single ventricle end of the spectrum is characterized by a severe degree of underdevelopment of the left heart-aorta complex, with a resulting inability of the left heart to support the systemic circulation. The hypoplasia of the left cardiac structures makes a biventricular approach unfeasible, which lead to the complex medical surgical management with a single ventricle multistage palliation and heart transplantation in specific situations.

7.3.2.1 Staged surgical palliation

The goal of staged reconstruction is creating separate pulmonary and systemic circulations supported by a single (right) ventricle. The Norwood procedure is usually the initial palliative procedure in the newborn, followed by a hemi-Fontan or bidirectional Glenn anastomosis (bidirectional cavopulmonary shunt) at 4-6 months and by a modified Fontan procedure (total cavopulmonary connection) at 2-4 years of age (Ashburn et al., 2003; Barron et al., 2009; Bove et al., 2004).

The Norwood procedure (Norwood et al., 1983) consists on atrial septectomy, reconstruction of the aortic arch to remove associated hypoplasia or coarctation, connection of the main pulmonary artery into this reconstructed arch and placement of a small shunt between the systemic and the pulmonary circulations achieved either by a Blalock-Taussig or by a Gore-tex shunt (the classical Norwood operation) or by a right ventricular to pulmonary artery conduit (the Norwood procedure with the Sano modification) (Sano et al., 2004). The Sano modification typically eliminates the diastolic runoff into the pulmonary circulation with subsequent coronary steal and potential risk of sudden death, with the limiting factor of limited pulmonary artery growth requiring performing the bidirectional cavopulmonary shunt earlier than what is required following the classical Norwood procedure. Early mortality of the first stage of palliation was very high (30-35%) in the first series but has dramatically improved, with current early survival of 80-90% (McGuirk et al., 2006; Stasik et al., 2006; Tweddell et al., 2002). Several operative risk factors have been identified including late initial presentation, prematurity, low birthweight (less than 3 kg), associated genetic anomalies, an ascending aorta smaller than 2 mm, intact or restrictive atrial septum, moderate or severe tricuspid regurgitation and pre-existing ventricular dysfunction (Ashburn et al., 2003; Azakie et al., 2001; Stasik et al., 2006; Tweddell et al., 2002). Although the Norwood operation remains one of the highest risk procedures in pediatric cardiac surgery, the second and third stages are much less hazardous, with 1-6% of early mortality (Gentles et al., 1997; Hirsch et al., 2008). Considering both peri-procedural and interstage mortality, actuarial survival after a Norwood procedure is 58-66% at 1 year (Ashburn et al., 2003; McGuirk et al., 2006; Tweddell et al., 2002), 40-61% at 5 years (Ashburn et al., 2003; Azakie et al., 2001; McGuirk et al., 2006; Tweddell et al., 2002) and 50% at 10 years (McGuirk et al., 2006). Long-term and functional outcome data following the staged univentricular palliation is being evaluated, with the expectation that these ventricles are likely to fail, on the basis of observations of other situations in which the right ventricle supports the systemic circulation, such as congenitally corrected transposition (Barron et al., 2009).

7.3.2.2 Cardiac transplantation

The concept of transplantation as a treatment for hypoplastic left heart syndrome developed together with the palliative approach of the Norwood procedure. Data from several centers show an 11-14% early mortality following the procedure (Chrisant et al., 2005; Razzouk et al., 1996), with a post-transplant actuarial survival of 84% (Razzouk et al., 1996), 72-76% (Chrisant et al., 2005; Razzouk et al., 1996) and 70% (Razzouk et al., 1996) at 1, 5 and 7 years, respectively. Innovations in peri-transplant management such as the development of new immunosuppressive strategies and the realization that ABO incompatibility is possible in neonatal transplantation because the immune response is not mature, have contributed to significantly improve its outcomes. Unfortunately, 20-25% of the patients die while awaiting for suitable donors (Jenkins et al., 2000; Razzouk et al., 1996), decreasing the rate of actuarial survival to 54-55% at 5 years when also accounting for these deaths (Chrisant et al., 2005; Jenkins et al., 2000). Although the benefit of a biventricular physiology produces better quality of life in children who receive a successful transplant compared with age-matched palliative-staged patients, major disadvantages of cardiac transplantation include high mortality on the waiting list as well as the immunosuppressant side-effects and morbidities. Some authors have suggested that cardiac transplantation may be offered to those patients at higher risk in staged surgery (Jenkins et al., 2000).

7.3.2.3 The hybrid procedure

The hybrid procedure has recently emerged as an innovative alternative to the Norwood operation (Akintuerk et al., 2002). This technique offers the advantage of avoiding cardiopulmonary bypass, cardioplegic arrest and circulatory arrest in the neonatal period. As infants are thought to be less vulnerable to postoperative myocardial and neurologic injury than neonates, this strategy may be associated with improved neurodevelopmental and functional outcomes (Akintuerk et al., 2002; Bacha & Hijazi, 2005; Galantowicz & Cheatham, 2005). The hybrid procedure, which involves both surgeons and interventional cardiologists, consists on placing bilateral pulmonary bands to limit flow to the lungs, implanting a stent in the *ductus arteriosus* and performing a balloon atrial septostomy (occasionally placing a stent). It is performed through a standard sternotomy but does not require cardiopulmonary bypass. The second step of the staged palliation is carried out as usual at 4-6 months. It will include both cavopulmonary shunt and aortic arch reconstruction, typically without full circulatory arrest to the brain. It has been advocated that it may have an overall survival advantage due to the fact that an in-series circulation (hybrid procedure) is more stable than a balanced circulation (Norwood procedure), and it might also have a role in stabilizing patients awaiting suitable cardiac donors (Bacha et al., 2006). On the other hand, complications such as stent migration and stent occlusion may occur, and the second stage of the palliation may be more extensive and complex thus carrying increased operative mortality. Finally, no consensus exists on the future of the hybrid approach. The potential benefits it offers may be weighted against the risks it carries.

7.4 Percutaneous aortic valve replacement

Percutaneous valve replacement is being developed. Although semilunar valve replacement has been successfully performed in adults for the aortic position and also in children for the pulmonary valve position, an aortic replacement during childhood seems to be more challenging technically due to sheath size, coronary artery blockage and potential mitral valve injury (Schneider et al., 2004). Anyway, percutaneous valve implantation is currently in development and may have a role on selected pediatric patients in the future.

7.5 Physical activity

Physical activity is not restricted in asymptomatic patients with mild aortic stenosis; these patients can participate in competitive sports. Patients with severe aortic stenosis should be restricted from all competitive athletic sports, while those with moderate aortic stenosis should avoid competitive sports that involve high dynamic and static muscular demands.

Other forms of exercise can be performed safely, but it is advisable to evaluate such patients with an exercise test before they begin an exercise or athletic program. Patients with treated aortic stenosis are restricted from competitive sports on the basis of subsequent residual gradients after intervention by the same criteria (Bonow et al., 2005).

7.6 Endocarditis prophylaxis

Endocarditis prophylaxis for the prevention of infective endocarditis was recommended in the past for any degree of valvar aortic stenosis and even in patients with normal functioning bicuspid aortic valve. Antibiotic prophylaxis is no longer indicated in these patients. This new guideline emphasizes that maintenance of optimal oral health and hygiene may reduce the incidence of bacteremia from daily activities and is more important than prophylactic antibiotics for a dental procedure. ACC/AHA recommendations are outlined in table 3 (Nishimura & ACC/AHA, 2008).

Prophylaxis against infective endocarditis is reasonable for the following patients at highest risk for adverse outcomes from infective endocarditis who undergo dental procedures that involve manipulation of either gingival tissue or the periapical region of teeth or perforation of the oral mucosa:
1. Patients with prosthetic cardiac valves or prosthetic material used for cardiac valve repair *(*Class *IIa; Level of Evidence B).*
2. Patients with previous infective endocarditis *(Class IIa; Level of Evidence B).*
3. Patients with CHD (Class IIa; Level of Evidence B): • Unrepaired cyanotic CHD, including palliative shunts and conduits. • Completely repaired congenital heart defect repaired with prosthetic material or device, whether placed by surgery or by catheter intervention, during the first 6 months after the procedure. • Repaired CHD with residual defects at the site or adjacent to the site of a prosthetic patch or prosthetic device (both of which inhibit endothelialization).
4. Cardiac transplant recipients with valve regurgitation due to a structurally abnormal valve *(Class IIa; Level of Evidence C).*
Prophylaxis against infective endocarditis is not recommended for nondental procedures (such as transesophageal echocardiogram, esophagogastroduodenoscopy, or colonoscopy) in the absence of active infection *(Class III; Level of Evidence B).*

Table 3. Current infective endocarditis prophylaxis recommendations of the ACC/AHA related to aortic valvar stenosis and bicuspid aortic valve (Nishimura & ACC/AHA, 2008).

8. References

Acar, P. (2006). Three-dimensional echocardiographic in congenital heart disease. *Arch Pediatr.*, Vol.13, No.1, (January 2006), pp. 51-56.

Akintuerk, H.; Michel-Behnke, I.; Valeske, K.; Mueller, M.; Thul, J.; Bauer, J.; Hagel, K.J.; Kreuder, J.; Vogt, P. & Schranz, D. (2002). Stenting of the arterial duct and banding of the pulmonary arteries: basis for combined Norwood stage I and II repair in hypoplastic left heart. *Circulation*, Vol.105, No.9, (March 2002), pp. 1099-1103.

Alekyan, B.G.; Petrosyan, Y.S.; Coulson, J.D.; Danilov, Y.Y. & Vinokurov AV. (1995). Right subscapular artery catheterization for balloon valvuloplasty of critical aortic stenosis in infants. *Am J Cardiol.*Vol.76, No.14, (November 1995), pp. 1049-1052.

Alexiou, C.; Chen, Q.; Langley, S.M.; Salmon, A.P.; Keeton, B.R.; Haw, M.P. & Monro, J.L. (2001). Is there still a place for open surgical valvotomy in the management of aortic stenosis in children? The view from Southampton. *Eur J Cardiothorac Surg*. Vol.20, No.2, (August 2001), pp. 239-246.

Alexiou, C.; McDonald, A.; Langley, S.M.; Dalrymple-Hay, M.J.; Haw, M.P. & Monro, J.L. (2000). Aortic valve replacement in children: are mechanical prostheses a good option? *Eur J* Cardiothorac *Surg*. Vol.17, No.2, (February 2000), pp. 125-133.

Alsoufi, B.; Karamlou, T.; Bradley, T.; Williams, W.G.; Van Arsdell, G.S.; Coles, J.G.; Smallhorn, J.; Nii, M.; Guerra, V. & Caldarone, C.A. (2006). Short and midterm results of aortic valve cusp extension in the treatment of children with congenital aortic valve disease. *Ann Thorac Surg*. Vol.82, No4, (October 2006), pp. 1292-1299.

Alsoufi, B.; Karamlou, T.; McCrindle, B.W. & Caldarone, C.A. (2007). Management options in neonates and infants with critical left ventricular outflow tract obstruction. *Eur J Cardiothorac Surg*. Vol.31, No.6, (Juin 2007), pp. 1013-1021.

Ashburn, D.A.; McCrindle, B.W.; Tchervenkov, C.I.; Jacobs, M.L.; Lofland, G.K.; Bove, E.L.; Spray, T.L.; Williams, W.G. & Blackstone, E.H. (2003). Outcomes after the Norwood operation in neonates with critical aortic stenosis or aortic valve atresia. *J Thorac Cardiovasc Surg*. Vol. 125, No.5, (May 2003), pp. 1070-1082.

Azakie, T.; Merklinger, S.L.; McCrindle, B.W.; Van Arsdell, G.S.; Lee, K.J.; Benson, L.N.; Coles, J.G. & Williams, W.G. (2001). Evolving strategies and improving outcomes of the modified norwood procedure: a 10-year single-institution experience. *Ann Thorac Surg*. Vol. 72, No.4, (October 2001), pp. 1349-1353.

Bacha, E.A.; Daves, S.; Hardin, J.; Abdulla, R.I.; Anderson, J.; Kahana, M.; Koenig, P.; Mora, B.N.; Gulecyuz, M.; Starr, J.P.; Alboliras, E.; Sandhu, S. & Hijazi, Z.M. (2006). Single-ventricle palliation for high-risk neonates: the emergence of an alternative hybrid stage I strategy. *J Thorac Cardiovasc Surg*.Vol.131, No.1, (January 2006), pp. 163-171.

Bacha, E.A. & Hijazi, Z.M. (2005). Hybrid procedures in pediatric cardiac surgery. *Semin Thorac Cardiovasc* Surg *Pediatr Card Surg Annu*. (2005), pp. 78-85.

Bacha, E.A.; Satou, G.M.; Moran, A.M.; Zurakowski, D.; Marx, G.R.; Keane, J.F. & Jonas, R.A. (2001). Valve-sparing operation for balloon-induced regurgitation in congenital aortic stenosis. *J Thorac Cardiovasc Surg*. Vol.122, No.1, (July 2001), pp. 162-168.

Badaruddoza, Afzal, M. & Akhtaruzzaman. (1994). Inbreeding and congenital heart diseases in a north Indian population. *Clin Genet* Vol.45, No.6, (June 1994), pp. 288-291.

Balmer, C.; Beghetti, M.; Fasnacht, M.; Friedli, B. & Arbenz, U. (2004). Balloon aortic valvoplasty in paediatric patients: progressive aortic regurgitation is common. *Heart* Vol.90, no.1, (January 2004), pp. 77–81.

Barron, D.J.; Kilby, M.D.; Davies, B.; Wright, J.G.; Jones, T.J. & Brawn, W.J. (2009). Hypoplastic left heart syndrome. *Lancet* Vol.374, No.9689, (August 2009), pp. 551-564.

Bassili, A.; Mokhtar, S.A.; Dabous, N.I.; Zaher, S.R.; Mokhtar, M.M. & Zaki, A. (2000). Risk factors for congenital heart diseases in Alexandria, Egypt. *Eur J Epidemiol.*Vol.16, No.9, (2000), pp. 805-814.

Basso, C.; Boschello, M.; Perrone, C.; Mecenero, A.; Cera, A.; Bicego, D.; Thiene, G. & De Dominicis, E. (2004). An echocardiographic survey of primary school children for bicuspid aortic valve. *Am J Cardiol.* Vol.93, no.5, (March 2004), pp. 661-663.

Baumgartner, H.; Hung, J.; Bermejo, J.; Chambers, J.B.; Evangelista, A.; Griffin, B.P.; Iung, B.; Otto, C.M.; Pellikka, P.A. & Quiñones, M; American Society of Echocardiography; European Association of Echocardiography. (2009). Echocardiographic assessment of valve stenosis: EAE/ASE recommendations for clinical practice. *Eur J Echocardiogr.* Vol.10, no.1, (January 2009), pp. 1-25.

Baumgartner, H.; Stefenelli, T.; Niederberger, J.; Schima, H. & Maurer, G. (1999). "Overestimation" of catheter gradients by Doppler ultrasound in patients with aortic stenosis: a predictable manifestation of pressure recovery. *J Am Coll Cardiol.*Vol.33, No.6, (May 1999), pp. 1655-1661.

Beekman, R.H.; Rocchini, A.P. & Andes, A. (1991). Balloon valvuloplasty for critical aortic stenosis in the newborn: Influence of new catheter technology. *J Am Coll Cardiol.* Vol.17, No.5, (April 1991), pp. :1172–1176.

Beekman, R.H.; Rocchini, A.P.; Crowley, D.C.; Snider, A.R.; Serwer, G.A.; Dick, M. 2nd & Rosenthal, A. (1988). Comparison of single and double balloon valvuloplasty in children with aortic stenosis. *J Am* Coll *Cardiol.* Vol.12, no.2, (August 1988), pp. 480-485.

Beroukhim, R.S.; Kruzick, T.L.; Taylor, A.L.; Gao, D. & Yetman, A.T. (2006). Progression of aortic dilation in children with a functionally normal bicuspid aortic valve. *Am J Cardiol.* Vol.98, No.6, (September 2006), pp. :828-830.

Bhabra, M.S.; Dhillon, R.; Bhudia, S.; Sethia, B.; Miller, P.; Stumper, O.; Wright, J.G.; De Giovanni, J.V.; Barron, D.J. & Brawn, W.J. (2003). Surgical aortic valvotomy in infancy: impact of leaflet morphology on long-term outcomes. *Ann Thorac Surg.* Vol.76, No.5, (November 2003), pp. 1412-1416.

Bondy, C.A.; Turner Syndrome Study Group. (2007). Care of girls and women with Turner syndrome: a guideline of the Turner Syndrome Study Group. *J Clin Endocrinol Metab.* Vol.92, No.1, (January 2007), pp. 10-25.

Bonow, R.O.; Carabello, B.A.; Chatterjee, K.; de Leon, A.C. Jr.; Faxon, D.P.; Freed, M.D.; Gaasch, W.H.; Lytle, B.W.; Nishimura, R.A.; O'Gara, P.T.; O'Rourke, R.A.; Otto, C.M.; Shah, P.M. & Shanewise, J.S; American College of Cardiology/American Heart Association Task Force on Practice Guidelines. (2008). 2008 focused update incorporated into the ACC/AHA 2006 guidelines for the management of patients with valvar heart disease: a report of the American College of Cardiology/American Heart Association Task Force on Practice Guidelines (Writing Committee to revise the 1998 guidelines for the management of patients with valvar heart disease). Endorsed by the Society of Cardiovascular Anesthesiologists, Society for Cardiovascular Angiography and Interventions, and

Society of Thoracic Surgeons. *J Am Coll Cardiol.* Vol.52, no.13, (September 2008), pp. e1-142.

Bonow, R.O.; Cheitlin, M.; Crawford, M. & Douglas, P.S. (2005). 36th Bethesda Conference: recommendations for determining eligibility for competition in athletes with cardiovascular abnormalties. Task Force 3: Valvar Heart Disease. *J Am Coll Cardiol.* Vol.45, No.8, (April 2005), pp. 1334–1340.

Botto, L.D., Correa, A. & Erickson, J.D. (2001). Racial and temporal variations in the prevalence of heart defects. *Pediatrics* Vol. 107, No. 3, (2001), pp. E32.

Bove, E.L.; Ohye, R.G. & Devaney, E.J. (2004). Hypoplastic left heart syndrome: conventional surgical management. *Semin Thorac Cardiovasc Surg Pediatr Card Surg Annu.* Vol. 7, (2004), pp. 3-10.

Brown, J.W.; Ruzmetov, M.; Shahriari, A.; Rodefeld, M.D.; Mahomed, Y. & Turrentine, M.W. (2009). Midterm results of Ross aortic valve replacement: a single-institution experience. *Ann Thorac Surg.* Vol.88, No.2, August 2009, pp. 601-607.

Brown, J.W.; Ruzmetov, M.; Vijay, P.; Rodefeld, M.D. & Turrentine, M.W. (2006). Closed transventricular aortic valvotomy for critical aortic stenosis in neonates: outcomes, risk factors, and reoperations. *Ann Thorac Surg.* Vol.81, No.1, (January 2006), pp. 236-242.

Brown, J.W.; Ruzmetov, M.; Vijay, P.; Rodefeld, M.D. & Turrentine, M.W. (2003). Surgery for aortic stenosis in children: a 40-year experience. Ann *Thorac Surg.* Vol.76, No.5, (November 2003), pp. 1398-1411.

Campbell, M. (1968). The natural history of congenital aortic stenosis. *Br Heart J.* Vol.30, no.4, (July 1968), pp. :514-526.

Cawley, P.J.; Maki, J.H. & Otto, C.M. (2009). Cardiovascular magnetic resonance imaging for valvar heart disease: technique and validation. *Circulation* Vol.119, No.3, (January 2009), pp. 468-478.

Champsaur, G.; Robin, J.; Tronc, F.; Curtil, A.; Ninet, J.; Sassolas, F.; Vedrinne, C. & Bozio, A. (1997). Mechanical valve in aortic position is a valid option in children and adolescents. *Eur J Cardiothorac Surg.* Vol.11; No.1, (January 1997), pp. 117-122.

Chang, A.C.; Huhta, J.C.; Yoon, G.Y.; Wood, D.C.; Tulzer, G.; Cohen, A.; Mennuti, M. & Norwood, W.I. (1991). Diagnosis, transport, and outcome in fetuses with left ventricular outflow tract obstruction. *J Thorac Cardiovasc Surg.*I Vol.102, No.6, (December 1991), pp. 841-848.

Chehab, G.; Chedid, P.; Saliba, Z. & Bouvagnet, P. (2007). Congenital cardiac disease and inbreeding: specific defects escape higher risk due to parental consanguinity. *Cardiol Young.* Vol.17; No.4, (August 2007), pp. 414-422.

Chrisant, M.R.; Naftel, D.C.; Drummond-Webb, J.; Chinnock, R.; Canter, C.E.; Boucek, M.M.; Boucek, RJ.; Hallowell, SC.; Kirklin, J.K. & Morrow, W.R.; Pediatric Heart Transplant Study Group. (2005). Fate of infants with hypoplastic left heart syndrome listed for cardiac transplantation: a multicenter study. *J Heart Lung Transplant.* Vol.24, No.5, (May 2005), pp. 576-582.

Chui, M.C.; Newby, D.E.; Panarelli, M.; Bloomfield, P. & Boon, N.A. (2001). Association between calcific aortic stenosis and hypercholesterolemia: is there a need for a randomized controlled trial of cholesterol-lowering therapy?. *Clin Cardiol.* Vol.24, No.1, (January 2001), pp. 52-55.

Clark, C. (1976). The fluid mechanics of aortic stenosis--I. Theory and steady flow experiments. *J Biomech.* Vol.9, No.8, (1976), pp. 521-528.

Clementi, M.; Notari, L.; Borghi, A. & Tenconi, R. (1996). Familial congenital bicuspid aortic valve: a disorder of uncertain inheritance. *Am J Med Genet.*Vol.62, No.4, (April 1996), pp. 336-338.

Cobanoglu, A. & Dobbs, J.L. (1996). Critical aortic stenosis in the neonate. Results of aortic commissurotomy. *Eur J Cardiothorac Surg.* Vol.10, No.2, (1996), pp. 116-119.

Corno, A.F.; Goy, J.J.; Hurni, M.; Payot, M.; Sekarski, N. & von Segesser, L.K. (2001). Treatment of congenital aortic valve stenosis: impact of the Ross operation. *Swiss Med Wkly.*Vol.131, No.5-6, (February 2001), pp. 65-69.

Cowley, C.G.; Dietrich, M.; Mosca, R.S.; Bove E.L.; Rocchini A.P. & Lloyd T.R. (2001). Balloon valvuloplasty versus transventricular dilation for neonatal critical aortic stenosis. *Am J Cardiol.* Vol.87, No.9, (May 2001), pp. 1125-1127.

Crespo, D.; Miró, J.; Vobecky, S.J.; Poirier, N.; Lapierre, C.; Zhao, N.N. & Dahdah N. (2009). Experience in a single centre with percutaneous aortic valvoplasty in children, including those with associated cardiovascular lesions. *Cardiol Young.* Vol.19, No.4, (august 2009), pp. 372-382.

Cripe, L.; Andelfinger, G.; Martin J.; Shooner, K. & Benson D.W. (2004). Bicuspid aortic valve is heritable. *J Am Coll Cardiol.* Vol.44, No.1, (July 2004), pp. 138-143.

Currie, P.J.; Seward J.B.; Reeder, G.S.; Vlietstra, R.E.; Bresnahan, D.R.; Bresnahan, J.F.; Smith,, H.C.; Hagler, D.J. & Tajik, A.J. (1985). Continuous-wave Doppler echocardiographic assessment of severity of calcific aortic stenosis: a simultaneous Doppler-catheter correlative study in 100 adult patients. *Circulation* Vol.71, No.6, (Juin 1985), pp. 1162-1169.

Daehnert, I.; Rotzch, C.; Wiener, M. & Schneider, P. (2004). Rapid right ventricular pacing is an alternative to adenosine in catheter interventional procedures for congenital heart disease. *Heart* Vol.90, No.9, (September 2004), pp. 1047-1050.

David, F.; Sánchez, A.; Yánez, L.; Velásquez, E.; Jiménez, S.; Martínez A. & Alva, C. (2007). Cardiac pacing in balloon aortic valvuloplasty. *Int J Cardiol.* Vol.116, No.3, (April 2007), pp. 327-330.

De Oliveira, N.C.; Ashburn,. D.A.; Khalid, F.; Burkhart, H.M.; Adatia, I.T.; Holtby, H.M.; Williams, W.G. & Van Arsdell, G.S. (2004). Prevention of early sudden circulatory collapse after the Norwood operation. *Circulation* Vol.110, No.11Suppl.1, (September 2004), pp. II133-138.

De Sa, M.; Moshkovitz, Y.; Butany, J. & David, T.E. (1999). Histologic abnormalities of the ascending aorta and pulmonary trunk in patients with bicuspid aortic valve disease: clinical relevance to the Ross procedure. *J Thorac Cardiovasc Surg.* Vol.118, No.4, (October 1999), pp. 588-194.

Edwards, J.E. (1965). Pathology of left ventricular outflow tract obstruction. *Circulation* Vol.31, (1965), pp. 586-599.

Elkins, R.C. (1999). Aortic valve: The Ross operation - a 12-year experience. *Ann Thorac Surg.* Vol.68, No.3Suppl., (September 1999), pp. 514-518.

El-Said, G.; Galioto, F.M. Jr.; Mullins, C.E. & McNamara, D.G. (1972). Natural hemodynamic history of congenital aortic stenosis in childhood. *Am J Cardiol.* Vol.30, no.1, (July 1972), pp. 6-12.

Falcone, M.W.; Roberts, W.C.; Morrow, A.G. & Perloff, J.K. (1971). Congenital aortic stenosis resulting from a unicommisssural valve. Clinical and anatomic features in twenty-one adult patients. *Circulation* Vol.44, No.2, (August 1971), pp. 272-280.

Fischer, D.R.; Ettedgui, J.A.; Park, S.C.; Siewers, R.D. & Del Nido, P.J. (1990). Carotid artery approach for balloon dilation of aortic valve stenosis in the neonate: A preliminary report. *J Am Coll Cardiol.* Vol.15, No.7, (Juin 1990), pp. 1633-1636.

Fowler, R.S.; Wood, M.M.; Bain, H.; Patel, R.G.; Sandor, G.G. & Rowe R.D. (1982). The ECG in aortic stenosis. Value of TAVF and QV6. *Pediatr Cardiol.* Vol.3, No.3, (1983), pp. 213-218.

Fratz, S.; Gildein, H.P.; Balling, G.; Sebening, W.; Genz, T.; Eicken, A. & Hess, J. (2008). Aortic valvuloplasty in pediatric patients substantially postpones the need for aortic valve surgerypp. a single-center experience of 188 patients after up to 17.5 years of follow-up. *Circulation* Vol.117, No.9, (Mars 2008), pp. 1201-1206.

Fyler, D.C. (1992). Aortic stenosis. In: Nadas´ Pediatric Cardiology, AS Nadas, DC Fyler (Eds.), pp. 493-51, Elsevier Health Sciences Publisher, ISBN 093288394X, Philadelphia.

Galal, O.; Rao, P.S.; Al-Fadley, F. & Wilson, A.D. (1997). Follow-up results of balloon aortic valvoplasty in children with special reference to causes of late aortic insufficiency. *Am Heart J.* Vol.133, No.4, (April 1997), pp. 418-427.

Galantowicz, M. & Cheatham, J.P. (2005). Lessons learned from the development of a new hybrid strategy for the management of hypoplastic left heart syndrome. *Pediatr Cardiol.* Vol.26, No.2, (March-April 2005), pp. 190-199.

Garg, V.; Muth, A.N.; Ransom, J.F.; Schluterman, M,K.; Barnes, R.; King, I.N.; Grossfeld, P.D. & Srivastava, D. (2005). Mutations in NOTCH1 cause aortic valve disease. *Nature* Vol.437, No.7056, (September 2005), pp. 270-274.

Gatrad, A.R.; Read, A.P. & Watson, G.H. (1984). Consanguinity and complex cardiac anomalies with situs ambiguus. *Arch Dis Child.*Vol.59, No.3, (March 1984), pp. 242-245.

Gatzoulis, M.A.; Rigby, M.L.; Shinebourne, E.A. & Redington, A.N. (1995). Contemporary results of balloon valvoplasty and surgical valvulotomy for congenital aortic stenosis. *Arch Dis Child.* Vol.73, No.1, (July 1995), pp. 66-69.

Gaynor, J.W.; Bull, C.; Sullivan, I.D.; Armstrong, B.E.; Deanfield, J.E.; Taylor, J.F.; Rees, P.G.; Ungerleider, R.M.; de Leval, M.R. & Stark. J. (1995). Late outcome of survivors of intervention for neonatal aortic valve stenosis. *Ann Thorac Surg.* Vol.60, no.1, (July 1995), pp. 122-125.

Gentles, T.L.; Mayer, J.E. Jr.; Gauvreau, K.; Newburger, J.W.; Lock, J.E.; Kupferschmid, J.P.; Burnett, J.; Jonas, R.A.; Castañeda, A.R. & Wernovsky, G. (1997). Fontan operation in five hundred consecutive patients: factors influencing early and late outcome. *J Thorac Cardiovasc Surg.* Vol.114, No.3, (September 1997), pp. 376-391.

Gersony, W.M.; Hayes, C.J.; Driscoll, D.J.; Keane, J.F.; Kidd, L.; O'Fallon, W.M.; Pieroni, D.R.; Wolfe, R.R. & Weidman, W.H. (1993). Bacterial endocarditis in patients with aortic stenosis, or ventricular septal defect. The Report of the Second Natural History Study of Congenital Heart Defects. *Circulation* Vol.87, No.2Suppl., (February 1993), pp. I121-126.

Gildein, H.P.; Kleinert, S.; Weintraub, R.G.; Wilkinson, J.L.; Karl, T.R. & Mee, R.B. (1996). Surgical commissurotomy of the aortic valve: outcome of open valvotomy in neonates with critical aortic stenosis. *Am Heart J.* Vo.131, No.4, (April 1996), pp. 754-759.

Glick, B.N. & Roberts, W.C. (1994). Congenitally bicuspid aortic valve in multiple family members. *Am J Cardiol.* Vol.73, No.5, (February 1994), pp. 400-404.

Gravholt, C.H. (2001). Aspects of the treatment of Turner syndrome. *Expert Opin Pharmacother.* Vol.2, No.10, (October 2001), pp. 1633-1647.

Gravholt, C.H. (2004). Epidemiological, endocrine and metabolic features in Turner syndrome. *Eur J Endocrinol.* Vol.151, no.6, (December 2004), pp. 657-687.

Gurvitz, M.; Chang, R.K.; Drant, S. & Allada, V. (2004). Frequency of aortic root dilation in children with a bicuspid aortic valve. *Am J Cardiol.* Vol.94, No.10, (Novemebr 2004), pp. 1337-1340.

Hausdorf, G.; Schneider, M.; Schirmer, K.R.; Schulze-Neick, I. & Lange, P.E. (1993). Antegrade balloon valvuloplasty of aortic stenosis in children. *Am J Cardiol.* Vol.71, No.5, (February 1993), pp. 460-463.

Hawkins.; J.A.; Minich LL.; Shaddy RE.; Tani LY.; Orsmond GS.; Sturtevant JE. & McGough EC. (1996). Aortic valve repair and replacement after balloon aortic valvuloplasty in children. *Ann Thorac Surg.* Vol.61, No.5, (May 1996), pp. 1355-1358.

Hawkins, J.A.; Minich, L.L.; Tani, L.Y.; Day, R.W.; Judd, V.E.; Shaddy, R.E. & McGough, E.C. (1998). Late results and reintervention after aortic valvotomy for critical aortic stenosis in neonates and infants. *Ann Thorac Surg.* Vol.65, No.6, (June 1998), pp. 1758-1762.

Hirsch, J.C.; Goldberg, C.; Bove, E.L.; Salehian, S.; Lee, T.; Ohye, R.G. & Devaney, E.J. (2008). Fontan operation in the current era: a 15-year single institution experience. *Ann Surg.* Vol.248, no.3, (September 2008), pp. 402-410.

Hoffman, J.I. & Kaplan, S. (2002). The incidence of congenital heart disease. *J Am Coll Cardiol.* Vol.39, no.12, (June 2002), pp. 1890-1900.

Holmes, K.W.; Lehmann, C.U.; Dalal, D.; Nasir, K.; Dietz, H.C.; Ravekes, W.J.; Thompson, W.R. & Spevak, P.J. (2007). Progressive dilation of the ascending aorta in children with isolated bicuspid aortic valve. *Am J Cardiol.* Vol.99, No.7, (April 2007), pp. 978-983.

Hossack, K.F.; Neutze, J.M.; Lowe, J.B. & Barratt-Boyes, B.G. (1980). Congenital valvar aortic stenosis. Natural history and assessment for operation. *Br Heart J.* Vol.43, No.5, (May 1980), pp. 561-573.

Hraska, V.; Photiadis, J. & Arenz, C. (2007). Open valvotomy for aortic valve stenosis in newborns and infants. In: *Multimedia Manual of Cardiothoracic Surgery;* doi:10.1510/mmcts.2006.002311, available from http://mmcts.ctsnetjournals.org/cgi/content/full/2007/0619/mmcts.2006.002311

Iwata, Y.; Imai, Y.; Shin'oka, T. & Kurosawa, H. (2008). Subaortic stenosis associated with systolic anterior motion. *Heart Vessels.* Vol.23, no.6, (November 2008), pp. 436-439.

Jenkins, P.C.; Flanagan, M.F.; Jenkins, K.J.; Sargent, J.D.; Canter, C.E.; Chinnock, R.E. & Vincent, R.N.; Tosteson AN, O'Connor GT. (2000). Survival analysis and risk factors for mortality in transplantation and staged surgery for hypoplastic left heart syndrome. *J Am Coll Cardiol.* Vol.36, no.4, (October 2000), pp. 1178-1185.

Jone, P.N. & Schowengerdt, K.O. Jr. (2009). Prenatal diagnosis of congenital heart disease. *Pediatr Clin North Am.* Vol.56, No.3, (June 2009), pp. 709-715.

Kahn, R.A.; Marin, M.L. & Hollier, L. (1998). Induction of ventricular fibrillation to facilitate endovascular stent graft repair or thoracic aortic aneurism. *Anesthesiology* Vol.88, No.2, (February 1998), pp. 534-536.

Kahn, R.A.; Moskowitz, D.M. & Marin, M.L. (2000). Safety and efficacy of highdose adenosine-induced asystole during endovascular AAA repair. *J Endovasc Ther.* Vol.7, No.4, (August 2000), pp. 292–296.

Karamlou, T.; Jang, K.; Williams, W.G.; Caldarone, C.A.; Van Arsdell, G.; Coles, J.G. & McCrindle, B.W. (2005). Outcomes and associated risk factors for aortic valve replacement in 160 children: a competing-risks analysis. *Circulation* Vol.112, No.22, (November 2005), pp. 3462-3469.

Keane, J.F.; Driscoll, D.J.; Gersony, W.M.; Hayes, C.J.; Kidd, L.; O'Fallon, W.M.; Pieroni, D.R.; Wolfe, R.R. & Weidman, W.H. (1993). Second natural history study of congenital heart defects. Results of treatment of patients with aortic valvar stenosis. *Circulation* Vol.87, No.2Suppl., (February 1993), pp. I16-27.

Khalid, O.; Luxenberd, C. & Sable, C. (2006). Aortic stenosis: the spectrum of practice. *Pediatr Cardiol.* Vol.27, No.6, (November-December 2006), pp. 661-669.

Kiraly, P.; Kapusta, L.; Thijssen, J.M. & Daniëls, O. (2003). Left ventricular myocardial function in congenital valvar aortic stenosis assessed by ultrasound tissue-velocity and strain-rate techniques. *Ultrasound Med Biol.* Vol.29, No.4, (April 2003), pp. 615-620.

Kitchiner, D.J.; Jackson, M.; Walsh, K.; Peart, I. & Arnold, R. (1993). Incidence and prognosis of congenital aortic valve stenosis in Liverpool (1960-1990). *Br Heart J.* Vol.69, No.1, *(January* 1993), pp. 71-79.

Kouchoukos, N.T.; Masetti, P.; Nickerson, N.J.; Castner, C.F.; Shannon, W.D. & Dávila-Román, V.G. (2004). The Ross procedure: long-term clinical and echocardiographic follow-up. *Ann Thorac Surg.*Vol.78, No.3, (September 2004), pp. 773-781.

Kusa, J.; Bialkowski, J. & Szkutnik, M. (2004). Percutaneous balloon aortic valvoplasty in children: early and long-term outcome. *Kardiol Pol.* Vol.60, No.1, *(January* 2004), pp. 48-56.

Lababidi, Z. (1983). Aortic balloon valvoplasty. *Am Heart J.* Vol.106, No.4Pt1), (October 1983), pp. 751-752.

Lababidi, Z.; Wu, J.R.; Walls, J.T.; Walls JT. (1984). Percutaneous balloon aortic valvoplasty: Results in 23 patients. *Am J Cardiol.* Vol.53, No.1, (January 1984), pp. 194-197.

Lambert, E.C.; Menon, V.A.; Wagner, H.R. & Vlad, P. (1974). Sudden unexpected death from cardiovascular disease in children. A cooperative international study. *Am J Cardiol.* Vol.34, No.1, (July 1974), pp. 89-96.

Landin-Wilhelmsen, K.; Bryman, I. & Wilhelmsen, L. (2001). Cardiac malformations and hypertension, but not metabolic risk factors, are common in Turner syndrome. *J Clin Endocrinol Metab.* Vol.86, no.9, (September 2001), pp. 4166-4170.

Levine, R.A.; Jimoh, A.; Cape, E.G.; McMillan, S.; Yoganathan, A.P. & Weyman, A.E. (1989). Pressure recovery distal to a stenosis: potential cause of gradient "overestimation" by Doppler echocardiography. *J Am Coll Cardiol.* Vol.13, No.3, (March 1989), pp. 706-715.

Lock, J.E. (1987). Evaluation and management prior to catheterization. In: *Diagnostic and interventional catheterization in congenital heart disease,* JE Lock, JF Keane, KE Fellows (Eds.), pp. 1-12, Kluwer Academic Publishers, ISBN-0-79238597-7, Norwell, MA.

Lofland, G.K.; McCrindle, B.W.; Williams, W.G.; Blackstone, E.H.; Tchervenkov, C.I.; Sittiwangkul, R. & Jonas, R.A. (2001). Critical aortic stenosis in the neonate: a multi-institutional study of management, outcomes, and risk factors. Congenital Heart Surgeons Society. *J Thorac Cardiovasc Surg*. Vol.121, No.1, (January 2001), pp. 10-27.

Mack, G. & Silberbach, M. (2000). Aortic and pulmonary stenosis. *Pediatr Rev*. Vol.21, No.3 (March 2000), pp. 79–85.

Makikallio, K.; McElhinney, D.B.; Levine, J.C.; Marx, G.R.; Colan, S.D.; Marshall, A.C.; Lock, JE.; Marcus, E.N. & Tworetzky, W. (2006). Fetal aortic valve stenosis and the evolution of hypoplastic left heart syndrome: patient selection for fetal intervention. *Circulation* Vol.113, No.11, (March 2006), pp. 1401-1405.

Manganaro, L.; Savelli, S.; Di Maurizio, M.; Perrone, A.; Tesei, J.; Francioso, A.; Angeletti, M.; Coratella, F.; Irimia, D.; Fierro, F.; Ventriglia, F. & Ballesio, L. (2008). Potential role of fetal cardiac evaluation with magnetic resonance imaging: preliminary experience. *Prenat Diagn*. Vol.28, No.2, (February 2008), pp. 148-156.

Marshall, A.C.; Tworetzky, W.; Bergersen, L.; McElhinney, D.B.; Benson, C.B.; Jennings, R.W.; Wilkins-Haug, L.E.; Marx, G.R. & Lock, J.E. (2005). Aortic valvuloplasty in the fetus: technical characteristics of successful balloon dilation. *J Pediatr*. Vol.147, No.4, (October 2005), pp. 535-539.

Masuda, M.; Kado, H.; Ando, Y.; Shiose, A.; Nakano, T.; Fukae, K.; Tanoue, Y. & Tominaga, R. (2008). Intermediate-term results after the aortic valve replacement using bileaflet mechanical prosthetic valve in children. *Eur J Cardiothorac Surg*. Vol.34, No.1, (July 2008), pp. 42-47.

Mazzitelli, D.; Guenther, T.; Schreiber, C.; Wottke, M.; Michel, J. & Meisner, H. (1998). Aortic valve replacement in children: are we on the right track? *Eur J Cardiothorac Surg*. Vol.13, No.5, (May 1998), pp. 565-571.

McElhinney, D.B.; Lock, J.E.; Keane, J.F.; Moran, A.M. & Colan, S.D. (2005). Left heart growth, function, and reintervention after balloon aortic valvoplasty for neonatal aortic stenosis. *Circulation* Vol.111, No.4, (February 2005), pp. 451-458.

McCrindle, B.W.; Blackstone, E.H.; Williams, W.G.; Sittiwangkul, R.; Spray, T.L.; Azakie, A. & Jonas, R.A. (2001). Are outcomes of surgical versus transcatheter balloon valvotomy equivalent in neonatal critical aortic stenosis? *Circulation* Vol.104, No.12Suppl.1, (September 2001), pp. I152-158.

McCrindle, B.W.; for the Valvoplasty and Angioplasty of Congenital Anomalies (VACA) Registry Investigators. (1996). Independent predictors of immediate results of percutaneous balloon aortic valvulotomy in Children. Valvoplasty and Angioplasty of Congenital Anomalies (VACA) Registry Investigators. *Am J Cardiol*. Nol.77, No.4, (February 1996), pp. 286–293.

McDonald, K. & Maurer, B.J. (1989). Familial aortic valve disease: evidence for a genetic influence? *Eur Heart J*. Vol.10, No.7, (July 1989), pp. 676–677.

McElhinney, D.B.; Marshall, A.C.; Wilkins-Haug, L.E.; Brown, D.W.; Benson, C.B.; Silva, V.; Marx, G.R.; Mizrahi-Arnaud, A.; Lock, J.E. & Tworetzky, W. (2009). Predictors of technical success and postnatal biventricular outcome after in utero aortic valvuloplasty for aortic stenosis with evolving hypoplastic left heart syndrome. *Circulation* Vol.120, No.15, (October 2009), pp. 1482-1490.

McGuirk, S.P.; Griselli, M.; Stumper, O.F.; Rumball, E.M.; Miller, P.; Dhillon, R.; de Giovanni, J.V.; Wright, J.G.; Barron, D.J. & Brawn, W.J. (2006). Staged surgical management of hypoplastic left heart syndrome: a single institution 12 year experience. *Heart* Vol.92, No.3, (March 2006), pp. 364-370.

Meliones, J.N.; Beekman, R.H.; Rocchini, A.P. & Lacina, D.J. (1989). Balloon valvoplasty for recurrent aortic stenosis after surgical valvulotomy in childhood: immediate and follow-up studies. *J Am Coll Cardiol.* Vol.13, No.5, (April 1989), pp. 1106-1110.

Miyamoto, T.; Sinzobahamvya, N.; Wetter, J.; Kallenberg, R.; Brecher, A.M.; Asfour, B.; & Urban, A.E. (2006). Twenty years experience of surgical aortic valvotomy for critical aortic stenosis in early infancy. *Eur J Cardiothorac Surg.* Vol.30, No.1, (July 2006), pp. 35-40.

Mizrahi-Arnaud, A.; Tworetzky, W.; Bulich, L.A.; Wilkins-Haug, L.E.; Marshall, A.C.; Benson, C.B.; Lock, J.E. & McElhinney, D.B. (2007). Pathophysiology, management, and outcomes of fetal hemodynamic instability during prenatal cardiac intervention. *Pediatr Res.* Vol.62, No.3, (September 2007), pp. 325-330.

Mookadam, F.; Thota, VR.; Garcia-Lopez, A.M.; Emani, U.R.; Alharthi, M.S.; Zamorano, J. & Khandheria, B.K. (2010). Unicuspid aortic valve in adults: a systematic review. *J Heart Valve Dis.* Vol.19, No.1, (January 2010), pp. 79-85.

Moore, P.; Egito, E.; Mowrey, H.; Perry, S.B.; Lock, J.E. & Keane, J.F. (1996). Midterm results of ballooon dilatation of congenital aortic stenosis. Predictors of success. *J Am Coll Cardiol.* Vol.27, No.5, (April 1996), pp. 257-263.

Mullins, C.E.; Nihill, M.R.; Vick, G.W. 3rd.; Ludomirsky, A.; O'Laughlin, M.P.; Bricker, J.T. & Judd, V.E. (1987). Double balloon technique for dilation of valvar or vessel stenosis in congenital and acquired heart disease. *J Am Coll Cardiol.* Vol.10, No.1, (July 1987), pp. 107-114.

Nabulsi, M.M.; Tamim, H.; Sabbagh, M.; Obeid, M.Y.; Yunis, K.A. & Bitar, F.F. (2003). Parental consanguinity and congenital heart malformations in a developing country. *Am J Med Genet A.* Vol.116A, no.4, (February 2003), pp. 342-347.

Nishimura, R.A.; Carabello, B.A.; Faxon, D.P.; Freed, M.D.; Lytle, B.W.; O'Gara, P.T.; O'Rourke, R.A. & Shah, P.M. (2008). ACC/AHA 2008 Guideline update on valvar heart disease: focused update on infective endocarditis: a report of the American College of Cardiology/American Heart Association Task Force on Practice Guidelines endorsed by the Society of Cardiovascular Anesthesiologists, Society for Cardiovascular Angiography and Interventions, and Society of Thoracic Surgeons. *J Am Coll Cardiol.* Vol.52, No.8, (August 2008), pp. 676-685.

Niwa, K.; Perloff, J.K.; Bhuta, S.M.; Laks, H.; Drinkwater, D.C.; Child, J.S. & Miner, P.D. (2001). Structural abnormalities of great arterial walls in congenital heart disease: light and electron microscopic analyses. *Circulation* Vol.103, No.3, (January 2001), pp. 393-400.

Norwood, W.I.; Lang, P. & Hansen, D.D. (1983). Physiologic repair of aortic atresia-hypoplastic left heart syndrome. *N Engl J Med.* Vol.308, No.1, (January 1983), pp. 23-26.

Odim, J.; Laks, H.; Allada, V.; Child, J.; Wilson, S. & Gjertson, D. (2005). Results of aortic valve-sparing and restoration with autologous pericardial leaflet extension in congenital heart disease. *Ann Thorac Surg.* Vol.80, No.2, (August 2005), pp. 647-654.

Otto, C.M.; Burwash, I.G.; Legget, M.E.; Munt, B.I.; Fujioka, M.; Healy, N.L.; Kraft, C.D.; Miyake-Hull, C.Y. & Schwaegler, R.G. (1997). Prospective study of asymptomatic valvar aortic stenosis. Clinical, echocardiographic, and exercise predictors of outcome. *Circulation* Vol.95, No.9, (May 1997), pp. 2262-2270.

Oury, J.H.; Hiro, S.P.; Maxwell, J.M.; Lamberti, J.J. & Duran, C.M. (1998). The Ross procedure: current registry results. *Ann Thorac Surg*. Vol.66, No.6Suppl., (December 1998), pp. S162-165.

Oury, J.H. (1996). Clinical aspects of the Ross procedure: indications and contraindications. *Semin Thorac Cardiovasc Surg*. Vol.8, No.4, (October 1996), pp. 328-335.

Pachulski, R.T.; Weinberg, A.L. & Chan, K.L. (1991). Aortic aneurysm in patients with functionally normal or minimally stenotic bicuspid aortic valve. *Am J Cardiol.* Vol.67, No.8, (April 1991), pp. 781-782.

Pedra, C.A.; Pedra, S.R.; Braga, S.L.; Esteves, C.A.; Moreira, S.M.; dos Santos, M.A.; Bosisio, I.J.; Silva, M.A.; Elias, P.F.; Santana, M.V. & Fontes, V.F. (2003). Short-and midterm followup results of valvoplasty with balloon catheter for congenital aortic stenosis. *Arq Bras Cardiol.* Vol.81.; No.2, (August 2003), pp. 120-128.

Phillips, R.R.; Gerlis, L.M.; Wilson, N.; & Walker, D.R. (1987). Aortic valve damage caused by operative balloon dilatation of critical aortic valve stenosis. *Br Heart J* Vol.57, No.2, (February 1987), pp. 168-170.

Polimenakos, A.C.; Sathanandam, S.; Blair, C.; Elzein, C.; Roberson, D. & Ilbawi, M.N. (2010). Selective tricuspidization and aortic cusp extension valvuloplasty: outcome analysis in infants and children. *Ann Thorac Surg*. Vol.90, No.3, (September 2010), pp. 839-846.

Popov, A.F.; Coskun, K.O.; Tirilomis, T.; Schmitto, J.D.; Hinz, J.; Kriebel, T.; Schoendube, F.A. & Ruschewski, W. (2009). Mechanical aortic valve replacement in children and adolescents after previous repair of congenital heart disease. *Artif Organs* Vol.33, No.11, (November 2009), pp. 915-921.

Poprawski, K.; Michalski, M.; Lawniczak, M. & Lacka, K. (2009). Cardiovascular abnormalities in patients with Turner syndrome according to karyotype: own experience and literature review. *Pol Arch Med Wewn.* Vol.119, No.7-8, (July-August 2009), pp. 453-460.

Rao, P.S.; Thapar, M.K.; Wilson, A.D.; Levy, J.M. & Chopra, P.S. (1989). Intermediate-term follow-up results ofballoon aortic valvoplasty in infants and children with special reference to causes of restenosis. *Am J Cardiol.* Vol.64, No.19, (December 1989), pp. 1356-1360.

Rao, P.S. (1999). Long-term follow-up results after balloon dilatation of pulmonic stenosis, aortic stenosis and coarctation of the aorta: a review. *Prog Cardiovasc Dis.* Vol.42, No.1, (July-August 1999), pp. 59-74.

Razzouk, A.J.; Chinnock, R.E.; Gundry, S.R.; Johnston, J.K.; Larsen, R.L.; Baum, M.F.; Mulla, N.F. & Bailey, L.L. (1996). Transplantation as a primary treatment for hypoplastic left heart syndrome: intermediate-term results. *Ann Thorac Surg*. Vol.62, No.1, (July 1996), pp. 1-7.

Reddy, V.M.; Rajasinghe, H.A.; Teitel, D.F.; Haas, G.S. & Hanley, F.L. (1996). Aortoventriculoplasty with the pulmonary autograft: The "Ross-Konno" procedure. *J Thorac Cardiovasc Surg*. Vol.111, No.1, (January 1996), pp. 158-167.

Reich, O.; Tax, P. & Marek, J. (2004). Long term results of percutaneous balloon valvoplasty of congenital aortic stenosis: independent predictors of outcome. *Heart* Vol.90, No.1, (January 2004), pp. 70-76.

Robbins, R.C.; Bowman, Jr. F.O. & Malm, J.R. (1988). Cardiac valve replacement in children: a twenty-year series. *Ann Thorac Surg.* Vol.45, No.1, (January 1988), pp. 56-61.

Roberts, W.C. & Ko, J.M. (2007). Clinical and morphologic features of the congenitally unicuspid acommissural stenotic and regurgitant aortic valve. *Cardiology* Vol.108, No.2, (2007), pp. 79-81.

Roberts, W.C. (1970). The congenitally bicuspid aortic valve. A study of 85 autopsy cases. *Am J Cardiol.* Vol.26, No.1, (July 1970), pp. 72-83.

Robida, A.; Folger, G.M. & Hajar, H.A. (1997). Incidence of congenital heart disease in Qatari children. *Int J Cardiol.* Vol.60, No.1, (June 1997), pp. 19-22.

Roos-Hesselink JW.; Schölzel BE.; Heijdra RJ.; Spitaels SE.; Meijboom FJ.; Boersma E.; Bogers AJ.; Simoons ML. (2003). Aortic valve and aortic arch pathology after coarctation repair. *Heart* Vol.89, No.9, (September 2003), pp. 1074-1077.

Ross, D.N. (1988). Pulmonary valve autotransplantation: the Ross operation. *J Card Surg.* Vol.3, No.3Suppl., (Septemebr 1988), pp. 313–319.

Ross, D.N. (1967). Replacement of the aortic and mitral valves with a pulmonary autograft. *Lancet* Vol.2, No.7523, (November 1967), pp. 956-958.

Rubio Vidal, M.D.; Deiros Bronte, L.; del Cerro Marín, M.J.; García Guereta, L.; Rodríguez R. & Moreno, F. (2008). Three-dimensional echocardiography: preliminary experience in congenital cardiac disease. *An Pediatr (Barc).*Vol.69, No.2, (August 2008), pp. 141-146.

Ruibal Francisco, J.L.; Sánchez Burón, P.; Piñero Martínez, E.; Bueno Lozano, G. & Reverte Blanc, F. (1997). Turner's syndrome. Relationship between the karyotypes and malformations and associated diseases in 23 patients. *An Esp Pediatr.* Vol.47, No.2, (August 1997), pp. 167-171.

Rychik, J.; Rome, J.J.; Collins, M.H.; DeCampli, W.M. & Spray, T.L. (1999). The hypoplastic left heart syndrome with intact atrial septum: atrial morphology, pulmonary vascular histopathology and outcome. *J Am Coll Cardiol.* Vol.34, No.2, (August 1999), pp. 554-560.

Samánek, M.; Benesová, D.; Goetzová, J. & Hrycejová, I. (1988). Distribution of age at death in children with congenital heart disease who died before the age of 15. *Br Heart J.* Vol.59, No.5, (May 1988), pp. 581-585.

Sano, S.; Ishino, K.; Kado, H.; Shiokawa, Y.; Sakamoto, K.; Yokota, M. & Kawada, M. (2004). Outcome of right ventricle-to-pulmonary artery shunt in first-stage palliation of hypoplastic left heart syndrome: a multi-institutional study. *Ann Thorac Surg.* Vol.,78, No.6, (December 2004), pp. 1951-1957.

Sarubbi, B.; Calvanese, R.; Cappelli Bigazzi, M.; Santoro, G.; Giovanna Russo, M. & Calabrò, R. (2004). Electrophysiological changes following balloon valvuloplasty and angioplasty for aortic stenosis and coartaction of aorta: clinical evidence for mechano-electrical feedback in humans. *Int J Cardiol.* Vol.93, No.1, (January 2004), pp. 7-11.

Schäfers, H.J.; Aicher, D.; Riodionycheva, S.; Lindinger, A.; Rädle-Hurst, T.; Langer, F. & Abdul-Khaliq, H. (2008). Bicuspidization of the unicuspid aortic valve: a new reconstructive approach. *Ann Thorac Surg.* Vol.85, no.6, (June 2008), pp. 2012-2018.

Schneider, D.J.; Levi, D.S.; Serwacki, M.J.; Moore, S.D. & Moore, J.W. (2004). Overview of interventional pediatric cardiology in 2004. *Minerva Pediatr.* Vol.56, No.1, (February 2004), pp. 1-28.

Shanmugam G.; MacArthur K.; Pollock J. (2005). Mechanical aortic valve replacement. Long-term outcomes in children. *J Heart Valve Dis.* Vol.14, No.2, (March 2005), pp. 166-171.

Shim, D.; Lloyd, T.R. & Beekman 3rd, R.H. (1997). Usefulness of repeat balloon aortic valvoplasty in children. *Am J Cardiol.* Vol.79, No.8, (April 1997), pp. 1141-1143.

Sholler, G.F.; Keane, J.F. & Perry, S.B. (1988). Balloon dilatation of congenital aortic valve stenosis. Results and influence of technical and morphological features on outcome. *Circulation* Vol.78, No.2, (August 1988), pp. 351-360.

Siu, S.C. & Silversides, C.K. (2010). Bicuspid aortic valve disease. *J Am Coll Cardiol.* Vol.55, No.25, (June 2010), pp. 2789-2800.

Snider, A.R. (1997). Quantification of aortic regurgitation. In: *Echocardiography in pediatric heart disease,* A.R. Snider (Ed.),180-186, Mosby, ISBN-978-1-4051-7401-5, St Louis, MO.

Spencer, F.C.; Neill, C.A. & Bahnson, H.T. (1958). The treatment of congenital aortic stenosis with valvotomy during cardiopulmonary bypass. *Surgery* vol.44, No.1, (July 1958), pp. 109-24.

Stasik, C.N.; Gelehrter, S.; Goldberg, C.S.; Bove, E.L.; Devaney, E.J. & Ohye, R.G. (2006). Current outcomes and risk factors for the Norwood procedure. *J Thorac Cardiovasc Surg.* Vol.131, No.2, (February 2006), pp. 412-417.

Subramanyan, R.; Joy, J.; Venugopalan, P.; Sapru, A. & Al Khusaiby, S.M. (2000). Incidence and spectrum of congenital heart disease in Oman. *Ann Trop Paediatr.* Vol.20, No.4, (December 2000), pp. 337-341.

Sybert, V. (1998). Cardiovascular malformations and complications in Turner syndrome. *Pediatrics* Vol.101, No.1, (January 1998), pp. 1-7.

Tribouilloy, C.; Avinée, P.; Shen, W.F.; Rey, J.L.; Slama, M. & Lesbre, J.P. (1991). End diastolic flow velocity just beneath the aortic isthmus assessed by pulsed Doppler echocardiography: a new predictor of the aortic regurgitant fraction. *Br Heart J* Vol.65, No.1, (January 1991), pp. 37-40.

Turner, C.G.; Tworetzky, W.; Wilkins-Haug, L.E. & Jennings, R.W. (2009). Cardiac anomalies in the fetus. *Clin Perinatol.* Vol.36, No.2, (June 2009), pp. 439-449.

Turrentine, M.W.; Ruzmetov, M.; Vijay, P.; Bills, R.G. & Brown, J.W. (2001). Biological versus mechanical aortic valve replacement in children. *Ann Thorac Surg.* Vol.71, No.5Suppl., (May 2001), pp. S356-360.

Tutar, E.; Ekici, F.; Atalay, S. & Nacar, N. (2005). The prevalence of bicuspid aortic valve in newborns by echocardiographic screening. *Am Heart J.* Vol.150, No.3, (September 2005), pp. 513-515

Tweddell, J.S.; Hoffman, G.M.; Mussatto, K.A.; Fedderly, R.T.; Berger, S.; Jaquiss, R.D.; Ghanayem, N.S.; Frisbee, S.J. & Litwin, S.B. (2002). Improved survival of patients undergoing palliation of hypoplastic left heart syndrome: lessons learned from 115 consecutive patients. *Circulation* Vol.106, No.12Suppl.1, (September 2002), pp. I82-89.

Tworetzky, W.; del Nido, P.J.; Powell, A.J.; Marshall, A.C.; Lock, J.E. & Geva, T. (2005). Usefulness of magnetic resonance imaging of left ventricular endocardial fibroelastosis in infants after fetal intervention for aortic valve stenosis. *Am J Cardiol.* Vol.96, No.11, (December 2005), pp. 1568-570.

Tzemos, N.; Therrien, J.; Yip J.; Thanassoulis, G.; Tremblay, S.; Jamorski, M.T.; Webb, G.D. & Siu, S.C. (2008). Outcomes in adults with bicuspid aortic valves. *JAMA.* Vol.300, No.11, (September 2008), pp. 1317-1325.

Villalba Nogales, J.; Herráiz Sarachaga, I.; Bermúdez-Cañete Fernández, R.; Maitre Azcárate, M.J.; Mora de Oñate, J. & González Rocafort, A. (2002). Balloon valvoplasty for critical aortic valve stenosis in neonates. *An Esp Pediatr.* Vol. 57, No.5, (November 2002), pp. 444-451.

Villavicencio, R.E.; Forbes, T.J.; Thomas, R.L. & Humes, R.A. (2003). Pressure recovery in pediatric aortic valve stenosis. *Pediatr Cardiol.* Vol.24, No.5, (September-October 2003), pp. 457-462.

Wagner, H.R.; Ellison, R.C.; Keane, J.F.; Humphries, O.J. & Nadas A.S. Clinical course in aortic stenosis. *Circulation* Vol.56, No.1Suppl., (August 1977), pp. I47-56.

Ward, C. (2000). Clinical significance of the bicuspid aortic valve. *Heart* Vol.83, No.1, (January 2000), pp. 81-85.

Warnes, C.A.; Williams, R.G.; Bashore, T.M.; Child, J.S.; Connolly, H.M.; Dearani, J.A.; del Nido, P.; Fasules, J.W.; Graham, T.P. Jr.; Hijazi, Z.M.; Hunt, S.A.; King, M.E.; Landzberg, M.J.; Miner, P.D.; Radford, M.J.; Walsh, E.P.; Webb, G.D.; Smith, S.C. Jr.; Jacobs, A.K.; Adams, C.D.; Anderson, J.L.; Antman, E.M.; Buller, C.E.; Creager, M.A.; Ettinger, S.M.; Halperin, J.L.; Hunt, S.A.; Krumholz, H.M.; Kushner, F.G.; Lytle, B.W.; Nishimura, R.A.; Page, R.L.; Riegel, B.; Tarkington, L.G.; Yancy, C.W.; American College of Cardiology; American Heart Association Task Force on Practice Guidelines (Writing Committee to Develop Guidelines on the Management of Adults With Congenital Heart Disease); American Society of Echocardiography; Heart Rhythm Society; International Society for Adult Congenital Heart Disease; Society for Cardiovascular Angiography and Interventions; Society of Thoracic Surgeons. (2008). ACC/AHA 2008 guidelines for the management of adults with congenital heart disease: a report of the American College of Cardiology/American Heart Association Task Force on Practice Guidelines (Writing Committee to Develop Guidelines on the Management of Adults With Congenital Heart Disease). *J Am Coll Cardiol.* Vol.52, No.23, (December 2008), pp. e1–121.

Weber, H.S.; Mart, C.R. & Myers, J.L. (2000). Transcarotid balloon valvuloplasty for critical aortic valve stenosis at the bedside via continuous transesophageal echocardiographic guidance. *Catheter Cardiovasc Interv.* Vol.50, No.3, (July 2000), pp. 326-329.

Weber, H.S. (2006). Catheter management of aortic valve stenosis in neonates and children. *Catheter Cardiovasc Interv.* Vol.67, No.6, (June 2006), pp. 947-955.

Wilkins-Haug, L.E.; Tworetzky, W.; Benson, C.B.; Marshall, A.C.; Jennings, R.W. & Lock, J.E. (2006). Factors affecting technical success of fetal aortic valve dilation. *Ultrasound Obstet Gynecol.* Vol.28, No.1, (July 2006), pp. 47–52.

Williams, I.A.; Quaegebeur, J.M.; Hsu, D.T.; Gersony, W.M.; Bourlon, F.; Mosca, R.S.; Gersony, D.R. & Solowiejczyk, D.E. (2005). Ross procedure in infants and toddlers followed into childhood. *Circulation* Vol.112, No.9Suppl., (August 2005), pp. I390-395.

Wolfe, R.R.; Driscoll, D.J.; Gersony, W.M.; Hayes, C.J.; Keane, J.F.; Kidd, L.; O'Fallon, W.M.; Pieroni, D.R. & Weidman, W.H. (1993). Arrhythmias in patients with valvar aortic stenosis, valvar pulmonary stenosis, and ventricular septal defect. Results of 24-hour ECG monitoring. *Circulation* Vol.87, No.2Suppl., (February 1993), pp. I89-101.

Zafra Anta, M.; Moreno Granado, F.; Calvo Rey, C.; Fernández Ruiz, A.; Rey del Castillo, C.; Cordovilla Zurdo, G. & Alvarez Díaz, F. (1993). Long-term results of surgical management of congenital aortic stenosis. *An Esp Pediatr.* Vol.38, No.3, (March 1993), pp. 213-219.

Zain, Z.; Zadinello, M.; Menahem, S. & Brizard, C. (2006). Neonatal isolated critical aortic valve stenosis: balloon valvuloplasty or surgical valvotomy. *Heart Lung Circ.* Vol.15, No.1, (February 2006), pp. 18-23.

2

Geriatric Aspects of Aortic Stenosis

Fatih Tufan, Fahrettin Öz, Ömer A Sayın and Hüseyin Oflaz
Istanbul University, Istanbul School of Medicine
Turkey

1. Introduction

There is a trend towards a worldwide aging in the last decades and diseases which are common in the elderly people would take important place in clinical practice. Aortic stenosis (AS) is a common and important condition among the elderly.

2. Etiology and prevalence

Currently, AS is the most frequent heart valve disease in industrialized countries and its prevalence sharply increases with age (Iung et al., 2003; Nkomo et al., 2006). Thus with the prolongation of life expectancy, the population of old patients with AS is expected to grow in the future. In elderly patients AS is most frequently caused by progressive calcification and degeneration of the tricuspid aortic cusps (Otto et al., 1997; Lindroos et al., 1994). The comissures are not fused as in rheumatic AS. Traditionally, AS has been thought of as a passive degenerative "wear and tear" disease associated with aging. Certain clinical factors like coronary artery disease (CAD), hypertension, obesity, diabetes mellitus, smoking, hyperlipidemia and chronic kidney disease (CKD) are associated with AS. However, the studies of Otto CM et al. support that the histopathological property of calcific aortic valve disease represents an active process with some similarities to atherosclerosis, including lipid deposition, macrophage and T cell infiltration, basement membrane disruption and microscopic calcification (Otto et al., 1994). Both AS and atherosclerosis have many clinical risk factors in common such as diabetes mellitus, hypertension, dyslipidemia, CKD, and tobacco use. (Peltier et al., 2003). Ortlepp JR et al observed that genetic factors may be important in the development of valve calcification (Ortlepp et al., 2001). They showed that patients with AS had significant difference in vitamin D receptor genotypes compared to individuals without AS.

The research of Stewart Bf et al. revealed that in 5201 men and women older than 65 years, 26% of study participants had frank aortic sclerosis (thickening of or calcific deposits on the aortic valve cusps with a peak velocity across the aortic valve of <1.5 msn) (Stewart et al., 1997). In the initial stages, aortic sclerosis is present without stenosis, but as the disease advances the valve leaflets which become less mobile eventually fuse together and cause left ventricular outflow tract (LVOT) obstruction. The study by Cosmi JE et al., in which more than 2000 patients with aortic sclerosis were examined, %16 developed AS (Cosmi et al., 2002). Of these patients mild, moderate and severe AS developed in 10.5, 3, and 2.5%

respectively. This cohort study showed that the average time interval of aortic sclerosis to AS was 8 years.
Other causes of AS in the elderly include rheumatic aortic valve disease (always occurs in conjunction with mitral valve involvement) and late degeneration of congenital bicuspid valves (Beppu et al., 1993; Pachulski et al., 1993). Congenital bicuspid valve anomaly accounts for about one fourth of AS in patients older 70 than years (Passik et al., 1987).

3. Pathopysiology

Regardless of the etiology, AS results in obstruction of LVOT. Obstruction of the LVOT leads to concentric hypertrophy (increase in LV wall thickness and mass) which normalizes systolic wall stress and maintains normal LV ejection fraction (LVEF) and cardiac output (Kennedy et al., 1968; Hood et al., 1968). Although hypertrophy helps to preserve ejection performance, it leads to abnormal LV compliance, LV diastolic dysfunction with reduced LV diastolic filling, increased LV end diastolic pressure and is associated with increased mortality (Levy et al., 1990; Zile et al., 2002). As the left ventricle becomes less compliant, atrial systole becomes more important for maintaining cardiac output, and onset of atrial fibrillation (AF) may result in clinical worsening and ventricular decompensation. The increases in systolic blood pressure, ventricular mass and ejection time lead to increased consumption of oxygen by the myocardium. Increased oxygen demand by the hypertrophic myocardium and abnormal patterns of coronary flow lead to angina pectoris in AS (Gould et al., 1997; Julius et al., 1997; Villari et al., 1992). Coexisting coronary disease is common with significant coronary narrowing in about 50% of elderly patients with AS (Georeeson et al., 1990). The increase in oxygen consumption and its contribution to decreased myocardial ischemia cause further deterioration of LV function. The stroke volume and cardiac output decrease and the mean left atrial and pulmonary capillary pressures increase and pulmonary hypertension occurs. This stage usually coincides with the occurrence of severe stenosis and the onset of symptoms. Several mechanisms have been postulated to explain the third cardinal symptom of AS, syncope. Although ventricular arrhythmias, bradyarrythmias and left ventricular systolic dysfunction have been proposed, most of the data suggests that an acute drop in blood pressure caused by inappropriate LV baroreceptor response because of increased LV pressures (Johnson et al., 1971; Richards et al., 1984).

4. Natural history

The patient with AS is generally asymptomatic for a prolonged period despite the obstruction and increased pressure load on the heart. Adults with asymptomatic AS have an excellent clinical outcome, indistinguishable from age-matched controls without aortic valve disease. It was estimated that sudden cardiac death accounted for 3-5% of all deaths in patients with asymptomatic AS (Braunwald, 1990). Hemodynamic progression in patients with AS has an average rate of increase in aortic jet velocity of 0.3 m/s per year, with an increase in mean transaortic pressure gradient of 7 mmHg per year and decrease in aortic valve area (AVA) of 0.1 cm^2 per year (Otto et al., 1989; Faggiano et al., 1996). However there is a wide range of hemodynamic progression among the patients with AS. Predictors of symptom onset in two studies included baseline jet velocity, the rate of change in jet velocity over time, the extent of valvular calcification, and functional status (Otto et al., 1997;

Rosenhek et al., 2000). The prognosis changes dramatically with the onset of symptoms of angina, syncope, or heart failure (HF) after a long latent period. The development of symptoms is a critical point in the natural history of AS. Older adults, who typically have decreased activity levels, experience delayed onset of clinical symptoms or they tend to relate their symptoms to other coexisting conditions. Ross and Braunwald found that the average survival after the onset of angina pectoris, syncope and HF was 3, 3 and 1.5-2 years respectively (Ross & Braunwald, 1968). In the study of Bouma et al., non-operated elderly patients with severe AS had a wide range of survival rates (Bouma et al., 1999). In this study, the three poor prognostic factors were a New York Heart Association (NYHA) functional class of III-IV, coexisting mitral regurgitation, and left ventricular systolic dysfunction. Survival was particularly poor (20% at 3 years) in the presence of NYHA III-IV symptoms and impaired left ventricle systolic function. The presence of AS in older adults increases their risk of having myocardial infarction and cardiovascular death (Aronow et al., 1998). Additional comorbidities which also affect survival are frequent in elderly patients with AS.

5. Symptoms

The cardinal manifestations of acquired AS are angina pectoris, syncope, and ultimately HF. Aranow et al. observed that in elderly patients, HF, syncope, or angina pectoris was present in 90%, 69% and 27% of patients with severe, moderate and mild AS respectively (Aranow et al., 1998). In the elderly, a clear description of the symptoms and their onset may be difficult to obtain. Most common initial symptom in the elderly is impaired exercise tolerance, exertional dyspnea and dizziness. In elderly symptoms of chest pain, shortness of breath, exercise intolerance, and dizziness are common and have many other potential causes, so that AS is generally not considered in the differential diagnosis. Symptoms may be absent in inactive elderly patient or may not be elicited from a patient with memory impairment. Establishment of symptomatic status and the severity of valvular disease can be troublesome because of subjectivity of symptom assessment and ambiguity of individual functional capacity in elderly (Sciomer et al., 2004). Concordantly, significant AS is underdiagnosed in the elderly.

Some patients may experience severe gastrointestinal bleeding secondary to angiodysplasia in association with AS (Heyde Syndrome, Bhutani et al., 1995). Infective endocarditis is less common in elderly patients with severe AS than in younger patients because endocardial surface is more calcific in the elderly. Endocarditic vegetations, AF and aortic atheromas represent important causes of systemic embolism including stroke in the elderly patients (Furberg et al., 1994; Tunick et al., 1994). Rarely, fragments of the calcific valve may embolize into the systemic circulation. Sudden death rarely occurs in asymptomatic patients. In the presurgical era, the incidence of sudden death in patients with symptomatic AS was estimated to be as high as 15-20% (Ross, 1968). Nowadays these rates decreased due to early surgical intervention in patients with symptomatic AS.

6. Signs

AS is often diagnosed after a systolic murmur elicited on physical examination necessitates an echocardiogaphic examination. Signs of AS include systolic ejection cresendo-decrescendo murmur that radiates to the neck and is often accompanied by a thrill. However, the murmur may radiate to the apex instead of the carotidis in elderly patients with AS (Gallavardin phenomenon). A prominent fourth heart sound (S_4) follows atrial systole in patients with sinus rhythm and noncompliant left ventricle. In the elderly, S_4 is less specific for AS, because hypertension, CAD, and other disorders which are common in older individuals can diminish left ventricular compliance (Lombard et al., 1987). In this setting, the physical examination findings of a soft murmur with an early peak, an upstroke of carotid impulse with normal timing, and a split second heart sound (S_2) suggest that mild or moderate AS is present. In a prospective study, carotid upstroke delay and amplitude, systolic murmur grade and peak, and a single S_2 predicted AS severity and clinical outcomes of death and symptom onset (Munt et al., 1999). On multivariate Cox regression analysis, the only physical examination finding which predicted the outcome was carotid upstroke amplitude. But most elderly patients with severe valve obstruction have only grade 2 or grade 3 murmur and some have an even softer murmur despite severe disease because of presence of concomitant HF or chronic lung disease (Lombard et al., 1987; Otto et al., 1997). The pulse pressure may be normal, or even wide, and the carotid upstroke may be rapid in the elderly with severe stenosis due to concomitant atherosclerosis of the arterial tree (Otto et al., 1997). So a slow rising, low amplitude carotid pulse has a relatively high specificity, but a low sensitivity, for the presence of severe AS in the elderly. No single physical examination finding or a combination of findings has both a high sensitivity and specificity for detection of severe AS. Older adults have an absent A_2 component of the S_2 due to aortic valve leaflet calcification which predominates with increasing age. Elderly patients with severe AS and aortic regurgitation have an A_2 component of the S_2, and in this situation, a soft diastolic murmur of aortic regurgitation may be heard.

7. Diagnostic tests

7.1 Electrocardiography

The ECG in patients with AS is not diagnostic. Findings of LVH are the most common findings on ECG in patients with severe AS. In the elderly patients, findings of LVH on ECG were seen in about two thirds of patients (Aronow et al., 1991). The voltage of the QRS complex may be markedly increased and ST-T wave changes which reflect chronic subendocardial ischemia are common. Other nonspecific signs include, left atrial enlargement, left axis deviation and left bundle branch block. AF can be seen at late stages and may otherwise suggest coexisting mitral valve disease or CAD.

7.2 Chest radiography

The chest radiography in AS is nonspecific. It is usually normal when AS is mild to moderate. Calcification the region of the aortic valve represents relevant chest radiography findings in the elderly, since calcific degeneration is the hallmark of AS in this age group. The radiographic features of compensated AS include concentric hypertrophy of the LV without cardiomegaly and poststenotic dilatation of the aorta. Of equal importance, the presence of cardiomegaly in a normotensive patient with isolated AS indicates decompensated AS.

7.3 Echocardiography

Doppler echocardiography is a cost–effective and accurate strategy to diagnose AS in the elderly (Otto et al., 1997). Echocardiography allows for the noninvasive assessment of the valvular structures and the real time evaluation of its hemodynamic consequences. It assesses left-ventricular functions, extent of hypertrophy, and amount of valve calcification. Standard evaluation of AS severity includes measurement of aortic velocity, mean transaortic pressure gradient, and continuity equation valve area (Figure 1). Anatomic images show the etiology of AS, level of obstruction, valve calcification, leaflet motion and aortic root anatomy. Echocardiography is also used to determine diastolic dysfunction by the presence of abnormal left ventricular relaxation. The velocity of blood flow increases as the stenotic orifice area decreases. Velocity measurements can be translated into pressure gradients across the aortic valve by using the Bernoulli equation. Aortic velocity allows classification of stenosis as mild (2.6-3 m/s), moderate (3 to 4 m/s), or severe (>4m/s). In case of leaflet thickening and calcification, presence of adequate leaflet motion and a velocity of <2.5 m/s defines aortic sclerosis. A mean aortic valve gradient greater than 40 mmHg on Doppler echocardiography is indicative of severe AS.

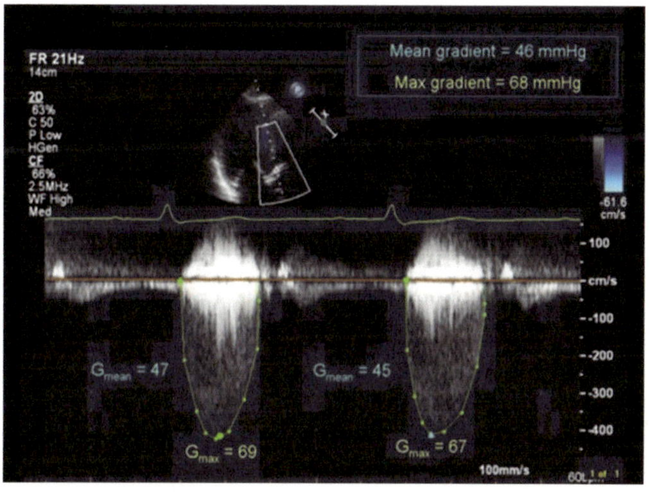

Fig. 1. To obtain the mean gradient, "trace" is used to trace the envelope of the aortic outflow. A mean aortic valve gradient greater than 40 mm Hg on Doppler echocardiography is indicative of severe AS.

The AVA can be estimated with the use of the continuity equation which depends on the principle of the law of continuity of flow (Carabello et al., 2003). Currently AS is graded as mild, moderate, and severe when the AVA is >1.5 cm^2, 1-1.5 cm^2, and <1 cm^2 respectively (Table 1). The most frequent error in measuring the AVA is due to the inaccuracy of LVOT diameter measurement. This is especially difficult in older adults in whom accumulation of calcium is present on the annulus. In order to avoid these errors some authorities suggest the use of dimensionless ratio for the assessment of AS. This index is simply the ratio of the velocity across the LVOT to the velocity across the aortic valve and completely eliminates the area of the LVOT from the equation (Otto et al., 2006). A ratio of 0.9-1 is accepted normal and a ratio of <0.25 indicates a valve area 25% of expected, corresponding to severe stenosis. Transesophageal echocardiography provides excellent short-axis images of the aortic valve, thus allows for direct measurement of the AVA by planimetry in many patients (Naqvi et al., 1999). Real time three dimensional transthoracic echocardiography offers an increased confidence level in the direct measurement of AVA (Vengala et al., 2004). Dobutamine stress echocardiography is often useful to estimate AVA and gradient at a higher cardiac output. It is particularly useful in patients with moderate to severe AS with low gradient and depressed LVEF. Truly severe AS shows only small changes (an increase of <0.2 cm^2) in AVA which remains <1 cm^2 with increasing flow rate but significant increase in gradients (mean gradient > 40 mmHg), whereas pseudosevere AS shows a marked increase in AVA with a final value of > 1 cm^2 but only minor changes in gradients. Dobutamine stress echocardiography also provides evidence of myocardial contractile reserve (increase of >20% of stroke volume during low dose dobutamine administration) (Vahanian et al., 2007; Bonow et al., 2006). Echocardiography is recommended to be performed yearly in patients with severe AS, every 2 years in patients with moderate AS, and every 5 years in patients with mild AS.

	Mild	Moderate	Severe
AoV_{max} (m/s)	2.5-3.0	3.0-4.0	>4.0
Peak gradient (mmHg)	<40	40-65	>65
Mean gradient (mmHg)	<20	20-40 (50)*	>40 (50)*
EOA (cont eq) (cm^2)	>1.5	1.0-1.5	<1.0
EOAi (cm^2/ m^2)	>0.85	0.60-0.85	<0.60
Dimensionless index	>0.50	0.25-0.50	<0.25

Table 1. Grading of aortic stenosis. *EAE guidelines only, otherwise both EAE and ASE.

7.4 Exercise testing

Severe AS is considered a contraindication for exercise testing (Ha, 2003). Nonetheless, in elderly patients with hemodynamically significant AS and ambiguous symptoms, exercise testing may be useful and safe if performed by an experienced physician. It is reasonable to perform the exercise testing it in patients over 70 years if they are still highly active. In asymptomatic patients, this test also may determine the recommended level of physical activity.

7.5 Cardiac catheterization

Its principle goal is to asses the extent of concomitant CAD (which is common in the elderly) by angiography rather than to determine the hemodynamic severity of AS. The valve should almost never be crossed, because the risk of death, stroke, or pulmonary edema is 7% if the valve is crossed and 3% for coronary angiography (Chambes, 2004). If the clinical findings are not consistent with the Doppler echocardiographic results, cardiac catheterization is recommended for further hemodynamic assessment. Cardiac catheterization should consist of the simultaneous measurement of the pressures in the left ventricle and in the aorta, enabling the calculation of the mean gradient. A "pull-back" tracing from the left ventricle to the aorta may be used in patients with normal sinus rhythm but it is not accurate in patients with rhythms disturbances or low-output states. In elderly patients with tortuous vessels the pull back technique may be preferred to a second femoral puncture needed to obtain a proper LV and proximal aortic pressure recording.

7.6 Computer tomography (CT)

Electron beam CT has the ability to detect and quantify calcification in AS (Pohle, 2004). It also allows detection of calcifications in coronary vessels and assessment of the ascending aorta (Pohle et al., 2004; Bouma et al., 1999). CT has shown high accuracy and reproducibility in quantifying aortic valve calcification and its progression. In patients with inadequate and inconclusive echocardiogram, CT may be as an alternative to obtain AVA.

7.7 Magnetic Resonance Imaging (MRI)

Cardiac MRI may be used to assess LV volume, function and mass. MR planimetry is reported to be highly reproducible and well tolerated and the results correlate very well with TEE results (Anna et al., 2003). Cardiac MRI is useful when acoustic windows in the echocardiogram are poor or when there is discordant imaging and catheterization results. It may also be an alternative to CT in patients with increased risk of contrast nephropathy because of older age and diminished baseline glomerular filtration rate (GFR).

8. Medical treatment

When symptoms of angina, syncope, or HF develop in patients with AS, the prognosis dramatically worsens. AVR represents the only proven treatment modality for symptomatic and hemodynamically significant AS. Other treatments such as medical therapy and TAVI are still controversial and researches are on way. There is no effective medical treatment for AS. Although medical therapy is unlikely to prolong survival, it may provide limited symptomatic relief. Hemodynamically significant AS is adversely affected by changes in preload and afterload. Potentially, all drugs used in symptomatic patients may cause worsening of the patients' conditions. Therefore, in patients with severe AS, drugs that reduce preload or afterload should be used with caution. In addition, due to the fact that chronic renal failure, autonomic dysfunction, and rhythm and conduction disturbances are more frequently seen in the elderly, side effects of drugs may be more dangerous.

8.1 Statins

Lipids are known to have important role in development of fibrosis and calcification seen in AS. Therefore, the use of lipid lowering drugs, especially the statins are recommended. Various studies suggested that the use of statins may reduce or prevent the worsening of fibrosis and calcification in patients with AS especially when used in the early periods. However, the results of the studies are conflicting and the effects of statins on the course of disease are not clear. Findings of several retrospective studies and at least one prospective trial show that patients receiving statins have slower progression of stenosis severity than do individuals not receiving them.(Rajamannan & Otto, 2004; Novaro et al., 2001). However, in a randomized trial of patients with moderate AS, Cowell and colleagues failed to show a benefit of high dose statin use in terms of halting the progression of valvular stenosis or inducing its regression (Cowell et al., 2005). Although the use of statins in patients with valvular AS is controversial, statins should be used in patients with AS and atherosclerotic vascular disease (Rossebø et al., 2008).

8.2 Angiotensin converting enzyme inhibitors (ACEI)

When patients with severe AS who can not tolerate AVR develop left HF symptoms, the use of ACEI may provide improvement in symptoms. Similar to statins, ACEI have been suggested to slow the progression of calcific valvular stenosis, but this suggestion has not been confirmed by findings of prospective studies (Rosenhek et al., 2004). On the other hand, the use of ACEI in patients with severe AS may increase the transvalvular gradient by reducing afterload or preload and may cause sudden deterioration of the patients' status. ACEI treatment should be initiated at low doses and gradually increased, avoidance of hypotension is crucial especially in the elderly patients.

8.3 Beta blockers

Beta blockers are not recommended for routine use. Patients with symptoms and signs of HF are not good candidates for beta blocker treatment because beta blockers may aggravate the symptoms of HF. Beta blockers are recommended for patients who experience angina pectoris or have AF with rapid ventricular response.

8.4 Diuretics

Diuretics are recommended in patients with lung congestion, ascites and edema. Diuretics provide improvement in HF symptoms by reducing left ventricular end-diastolic pressure. Diuretics should be used with caution because a low preload may exacerbate symptoms due to low cardiac output. Elderly patients may not excrete free water as efficiently as younger people do, and they may be more prone to develop hyponatremia after diuretic treatment (Clark et al., 1994). Thiazide diuretics are more commonly associated with hyponatremia than loop diuretics (Hwang & Kim, 2010). Nocturia is frequently seen in elderly patients and disruption of normal circadian rhythm of antidiuretic hormone may be an important factor in this issue (Moon et al., 2004). Elderly patients are also more prone to diuretic induced hyponatremia, because concomitant use of other medications like selective serotonin reuptake inhibitors (SSRI), which may precipitate hyponatremia, is common. Diuretics also lead to orthostatic hypotension by inducing volume depletion. Because falls are more frequent and are associated with greater morbidity and mortality in the elderly patients, monitoring of blood pressure at home and avoidance of hypotension is crucial. Evening and night doses of diuretics are also associated with more frequent nocturia and may increase the risk of falls during night. Thus, administration of diuretics in earlier hours may be safer.

8.5 Nitrates

Nitrates may be used in patients with severe AS who experience angina pectoris. Because it may cause sudden hypotension, it should be initiated at low doses and gradually increased. Concomitant use of nitrates with phosphodiesterase inhibitors, which are commonly used in the elderly patients with erectile dysfunction, should be avoided to prevent substantial hypotension.

8.6 Digoxin

Digoxin has a narrow therapeutic index and elderly patients may be more prone to side effects associated with its use (Cheng & Nayar, 2009). Digoxin is eliminated by the kidneys and impairment of kidney functions with aging is an important issue in this context. The recent ACC/AHA guideline recommends an initial dose of 0.125 mg daily or every other day if the patient is more than 70 years old, has impaired kidney function, or has a low lean body mass (Hunt et al., 2009). Using a target drug concentration of 0.5-1 ng/ml is recommended despite conventional therapeutic serum concentration is defined as 0.8-2 ng/ml (Hunt et al., 2009). A digoxin concentration above 1 ng/ml may not be more effective in terms of symptomatic relief and may potentially be associated with increased morbidity and mortality (Cheng & Nayar, 2009; Hunt et al., 2009). When hypokalemia, hypomagnesemia or hypothyroidism coexists, digoxin toxicity may occur with lower digoxin concentrations (Hunt et al., 2009). Elderly patients may also be more prone to develop adverse effects of digoxin like anorexia, nausea, vomiting, confusion, visual problems, and rhythm and conduction disturbances (Cheng & Nayar, 2009). Concomitant use of drugs which may interact with digoxin may also be common in the elderly. In this context, clarithromycin, erythromycin, amiodarone, itraconazole, cyclosporine, verapamil, and quinidine can increase serum digoxin concentrations (Hunt et al., 2009). The use of digoxin is contraindicated in patients with severe AS and sinus rhythm. When AF with rapid ventricular response and hemodynamic deterioration is present, digoxin may be used to reduce the ventricular rate. Because beta blockers improve survival in patients with HF and may effectively control heart rate alone, digoxin which is associated with aforementioned potential harms, should be used with caution as an adjunctive agent for heart rate control.

9. Perioperative evaluation and management

9.1 Evaluation and management

Decision to identify patients who are at high risk for cardiac surgery is cumbersome. This issue may be further complicated in the elderly. Some risk score algorithms like Ambler score, logistic EuroSCORE and Society of Thoracic Surgeons Predicted Risk of Mortality (STS-PROM) are widely used to identify patients at high risk for cardiac surgery. Ambler score was dedicated to predict in-hospital mortality after heart valve surgery (Ambler et al., 2005). EuroSCORE integrates increased age, female gender, chronic pulmonary disease, extracardiac arteriopathy, neurological dysfunction, previous cardiac surgery, increased serum creatinine, active endocarditis, critical perioperative state, unstable angina, LV dysfunction, recent MI, and pulmonary hypertension as patient and cardiac related factors and some operation related factors like emergency, other than isolated CABG, surgery on thoracic aorta, and postinfarct septal rupture (Nashef et al., 1999). An online calculator is available in their official website (http://www.euroscore.org/). The STS-PROM risk scoring which is more complicated integrates age, gender, race, weight, creatinine level, various chronic cardiac and non-cardiac diseases, previous cardiovascular interventions, perioperative cardiac status, hemodynamic status, and operative risk factors. This scoring estimates the rates of postoperative morbidity, mortality, permanent stroke, prolonged ventilation, renal failure, and reoperation. It is updated regularly and calculation can be performed only via the online calculator (http://www.sts.org/). Recent data indicates that these scores may also predict hospital charges and resource use (Arnaoutakis et al., 2011).

These risk score algorithms are widely used and validated, but they are not perfect and have many limitations (Rosenhek et al., 2011). Elderly patients above 75 years old constituted a small proportion of the cohorts used in these risk scores, thus extrapolation of these results to frail elderly patients who are generally above 75 years old may not give accurate results. In this context, a recent study which involved 1245 elderly patients (mean age 77.2 years) who underwent AVR with or without additional bypass surgery, suggested that among these three risk scores, only STS-PROM was correlated with operative mortality (Frilling et al., 2010). The authors emphasized that risk scores aimed specifically at geriatric patients might be necessary to accurately identify patients with high surgical risk. These scores have mainly been validated in patients undergoing CABG surgery, compromising their accuracy in patients undergoing heart valve replacement surgery (Rosenhek et al., 2011). Comorbidities not included in these algorithms may increase the risk of surgery. Rosenhek et al suggest necessity of including additional variables like cognitive and functional capacity to the risk assessment tools (Rosenhek et al., 2011). Moreover, the weighting of the risk factors are variable between these algorithms. For example, EuroSCORE includes a cutoff point for creatinine (200 μmol/L), which means a creatinine level above this level increases the risk, whereas a lower level does not increase the risk. This suggestion has two limitations. First, a creatinine level above this threshold in a 65 year old male who weights 90 kg may suggest a better renal function than a creatinine level below this level in an 85 year old female who weights 50 kg. Furthermore, the creatinine level may not reflect glomerular filtration rate (GFR) accurately in a slim and sarcopenic elderly patient. Pulmonary arterial systolic pressure is also categorized in a binary fashion, thus decreasing the value of this important risk factor in this scoring system. STS-PROM does not use a cutoff for creatinine level and utilizes creatinine level as a continuous variable. However, the muscle mass is an important determinant of creatinine levels. A low muscle mass may actually represent a poor prognostic factor while it would be associated with a lower creatinine level, thus decreasing the STS-PROM risk score. Using more accurate estimations of GFR like Cockcroft-Gault formula may give more important prognostic information. Cystatin C which is not influenced by muscle mass may potentially reflect GFR more accurately and its level increase in earlier stages of kidney insufficiency compared to creatinine. However, there are limitations with measurement techniques of cystatin C and estimation of GFR by cystatin C levels is not standardized because there are many cystatin C based formulas to estimate GFR. The physiologic changes associated with aging should always be considered. A comprehensive geriatric assessment would also provide invaluable information in the preoperative evaluation and postoperative follow up of the elderly patients.

Morbidity and mortality rates may also be influenced by other factors like experience of the surgeon and the center (Rosenhek et al., 2011). Thus it would be logical to compare local outcomes with those predicted by the risk scores. Nonetheless, the decision of an experienced physician or of a specialized team may be more accurate than the risk scores. A recent trial which utilized STS-PROM, presence of pulmonary hypertension, presence of porcelain aorta and the decision of the medical team that the patient is frail as the criteria to decide a patient is inoperable and to enroll them to TAVI procedures (Rodés-Cabau el al., 2010). They suggested that frail patients even with a low STS-PROM score had increased risk. Although the decision of an experienced medical team that a patient is frail may be accurate, usage of widely used criteria to identify frailty may be more accurate and enable utilization of frailty as a risk factor in the preoperative evaluation in a standardized manner.

Brain natriuretic peptide (BNP) is widely used for prognostic prediction in heart diseases. BNP is higher in symptomatic patients compared to asymptomatic patients (Carabello & Paulus, 2009). BNP may also predict onset of symptoms when elevated values are found in an asymptomatic patient and facilitate advising surgery to an asymptomatic patient with AS (Carabello & Paulus, 2009). Recently Monin et al. followed up 107 asymptomatic patients with moderate to severe AS to predict death or need for AVR and to build a continuous risk score using the independent predictors of this outcome (Monin et al., 2009). One of the most powerful predictors of outcome was BNP in this study. BNP levels were shown to predict postoperative survival and complications (Bergler-Klein et al., 2004; Nozohoor el al., 2009; Pedrazzini et al., 2008). Limitations of utilizing BNP include absence of a standardized cutoff for prediction of outcome in AS, interference of the predictive value of BNP with presence of renal dysfunction, pulmonary hypertension and obesity (Carabello & Paulus, 2009). Unlike BNP, amino terminal-proBNP levels may increase significantly when renal dysfunction exists, thus it seems more suitable to use BNP levels in patients with renal dysfunction (Tagore et al., 2008). Bernstein et al. suggest adjustment of proBNP levels with a formula utilizing estimated GFR level and age (Bernstein et al., 2009).

Sündermann at al utilized a comprehensive assessment of frailty (CAF) score to predict outcomes after cardiac interventions (CABG, valve surgery, TAVI or combined procedures) in 400 patients aged ≥74 years (Sündermann at al., 2011). This score integrated weakness assessed with grip strength, self-reported exhaustion assessed with a questionnaire, slowness of gait speed measured with 4 meter usual gait speed test, activity level evaluated by instrumental activities of daily living, standing balance, body control, forced expiratory volume in 1 s, and levels of albumin, creatinine, and BNP. Although the variables were used in a binary fashion in this study CAF score was found to be correlated with EuroSCORE and STS-PROM scores and also predicted 30-day mortality.

A recent study which investigated influence of preoperative LV diastolic functions on development of postoperative LV systolic dysfunction showed that besides advanced age and prolonged myocardial ischemic time, preoperative LV diastolic dysfunction was also an important determinant of LV systolic dysfunction after AVR operation (Licker et al., 2010). Another recent study assessed presence and degree of myocardial fibrosis on the outcomes after AVR (Weidemann et al., 2009). Intraoperative myocardial biopsy and preoperative and postoperative cardiac MRI were used to assess myocardial fibrosis in this study. They found a significant correlation of myocardial fibrosis with NHYA class and markers of longitudinal systolic function but not with global ejection fraction or aortic valve area. They found significant correlations between the presence and degree of myocardial fibrosis and clinical outcomes. Another recent study evaluated the influence of preoperative illness beliefs on postoperative disability, physical functioning, psychological well being and depressive symptoms (Juergens et al., 2010). Postoperative outcomes were correlated with patients' preoperative beliefs but not with cardiac risk factors used in this study (EuroSCORE and LVEF).

Spirometric pulmonary functions were assessed preoperatively in a recent trial and percentage of predictive forced vital capacity was found to be an independent predictor of in-hospital mortality, even when adjusted for the logistic EuroSCORE (Nissinen et al., 2009). They also suggested that this parameter was an independent predictor of postoperative stroke.

Preoperative six minute walk test with a cutoff value of 300 meters was utilized in patients undergoing AVR in a recent trial (de Arenaza et al., 2010). It was indicated that six minute walk test added prognostic information to EuroSCORE and was an independent predictor of the composite outcome of death, myocardial infarction or stroke at 12 months.

Monin et al suggested that a good outcome after AVR may be seen when severe AS caused left-ventricular dysfunction, especially if inotropic reserve is present (Monin et al., 2003). They utilized dobutamine stress Doppler hemodynamics to show presence of LV contractile reserve in their study.

Aside from a high risk score, there are some other factors like patient refusal and porcelain aorta which deem some of the patients inoperable. The opinion of the experienced physician is also important to define patients at higher risk for surgery and to provide required precautions for the patients. Furthermore there are more non-invasive procedures like TAVI which may be used in patients with a high surgical risk.

Current ESC and ACC/AHA guidelines were published in 2007 and 2008 respectively. ESC guidelines emphasize that AS is increasingly observed in the elderly and AVR could prolong and improve the quality of life despite the increased risks of morbidity and mortality in this population (Vahanian et al., 2007). It is also noticed that a large percentage of suitable candidates for AVR are not referred for surgery. It is recommended that age, per se, should not be considered a contraindication for surgery and decisions should be made on an individual basis, provided that patients' wishes and cardiac and non-cardiac factors are taken into account. It is also denoted that early intervention at an asymptomatic stage should be avoided. ACC/AHA guidelines state that no effective medical treatment exists and balloon valvotomy is not a suitable alternative to surgery (Bonow et al., 2008). Among denotations about valve surgery in elderly patients in these guidelines are: CAD and LV dysfunction are associated with worse outcomes; advanced diseases like cancer, stroke and dementia render surgery inappropriate; and deconditioned and debilitated patients often do not return to an active life after surgery. Other peculiar considerations stated for the elderly are: a narrow LVOT and a small aortic annulus could require enlargement of the annulus, heavy calcification may require debridement, and a composite valve-aortic graft may be needed. Importance of recognition of marked LV hypertrophy which could be a marker of perioperative morbidity and mortality is emphasized. Absence of a perfect method to weigh all of the relevant factors and to identify high- and low-risk elderly is also noted.

Data about comparison of mechanical prostheses and bioprostheses for AVR in the elderly is scarce. One recent report suggests good outcomes of bioprostheses for AVR after more than 10 years of follow up in the elderly (Suojaranta-Ylinen et al., 2009). In the Veterans Affairs randomized trial, patients who underwent single AVR or mitral valve replacement with mechanical valve versus bioprosthesis were enrolled in a randomized fashion (Hammermeister et al., 2000). They found a better survival with mechanical valves largely because primary valve failure was virtually absent in this the mechanical valve group while it was seen in an important proportion of the bioprosthesis group. However primary valve failure was not significantly different between these groups in the elderly population. While the rate of thromboembolism was similar between the groups, bleeding complications were more common in the mechanical valve group. It is of note that lifelong warfarin treatment is required in patients who undergo AVR with mechanical valves and bleeding complications with warfarin is more common in the elderly. Further trials are needed to compare the outcomes of AVR with mechanical valves and bioprostheses in the elderly.

Patients with severe AS may have markedly reduced platelet functions and thus experience increased postoperative blood loss. One recent double-blind placebo controlled trial investigated effects of infusion of desmopressin (0.3 μg/kg) on platelet functions and postoperative blood loss (Steinlechner et al., 2011). They recommended assessing of platelet functions and usage of desmopressin to avoid increased blood loss in patients with reduced platelet functions.

Among perioperative cautions for the patient with AS, careful manipulation of hemodynamics is crucial (Frogel & Galusca, 2010). Main goals to decrease the perioperative cardiovascular risk are to maintain sinus rhythm, a relatively slow heart rate, and adequate preload and afterload (Frogel & Galusca, 2010). In this context, a slower heart rate decreases myocardial oxygen demand and increases coronary perfusion time. Routine antibiotic prophylaxis is not recommended unless the patient has a previous history of infective endocarditis (Frogel & Galusca, 2010). Regarding anesthetic premedication, anticholinergics may cause tachycardia in a dose dependent manner and careful titration of sedation is crucial because oversedation may cause hypotension and undersedation may increase the sympathetic tone (Frogel & Galusca, 2010). Because of the risk of serious arrhythmias, a defibrillator should be readily available and placed on the patient before sterile draping. Ideal heart rate is in the range of 60 to 70 beats per minute and bradicardia should be avoided especially in the elderly patients who may have predisposition to it (Frogel & Galusca, 2010). As atrial systole is necessary for maximal LV preload, maintenance of normal sinus rhythm is very important. Adequate hydration is very important as well, since patients with AS are preload dependent (Frogel & Galusca, 2010). Elderly patients and patients with central nervous system disorders affecting sensation of thirst have tendency to develop dehydration and need careful evaluation of hydration status. Regarding type of anesthesia, an epidural technique may be preferred to neuroaxial anesthesia with sympathectomy because it allows incremental dosing and does not cause sudden changes in systemic vascular resistance (Frogel & Galusca, 2010). Opioids, midazolam, etomidate and cisatracurium may be good options for general anesthesia because they offer relatively stable hemodynamic effects (Frogel & Galusca, 2010). Careful monitoring of the blood pressure is pivotal and hypotension should be avoided and once hypotension develops it should be controlled with pure α agonists since they do not cause tachycardia (Frogel & Galusca, 2010). Invasive arterial blood pressure and central venous pressure monitoring are also recommended.

Elderly patients are at increased risk for experiencing adverse events like delirium and electrolyte disorders in the postoperative period. There are many metabolic, infectious and psychological factors which predispose the frail elderly to develop delirium. It is of note that delirium is very common after cardiac surgery and is associated with increased risk of short and long term morbidity and mortality (Maldonado et al., 2009). Psychotic symptoms of delirium like hallucinations and delusions are easily recognized, but many patients do not have these symptoms and routine assessment of attention and orientation is crucial. Of note, symptoms of delirium wax and wane and make identification of it difficult. Despite its high prevalence and adverse outcomes, many physicians do not recognize delirium (Maldonado et al., 2009). Giltay et al., focused on the psychotic symptoms of delirium after cardiac surgery and suggested that they are independently associated with adverse outcomes (Giltay et al., 2006). They found higher age, renal failure, dyspnea, HF, and left ventricle hypertrophy as independent preoperative predisposing factors and hypothermia (<33,8°C), hypoxemia, low hematocrit, renal failure, increased sodium, infection and stroke as independent precipitating factors. Careful monitorization of volume status, follow up of renal functions and electrolyte levels, adequate pain control and rational medication selection are of great importance. Many drugs like anticholinergics, antihistaminics,

narcotics and central acting drugs like benzodiazepines may precipitate delirium in an elderly patient with predisposing factors. When a precipitating factor for delirium is identified in a delirious patient, search of other potential causes of it should continue, because especially patients without dementia do not easily develop delirium. Maldonado et al. investigated the effects of postoperative sedation on the development of delirium in patients undergoing cardiac valve surgery (Maldonado et al., 2009). They compared dexmedetomidine, which is not a GABAergic agent, has no anticholinergic effects, promotes a more physiological sleep pattern without significant respiratory depression, and may be associated with a decreased need for opioid use, with current postoperative sedation practices (propofol or midazolam) in a prospective, randomized and open label trial. They showed a significantly decreased rate of delirium with dexmedetomidine compared to propofol and midazolam (rates of delirium 3%, 50% and 50% respectively).
Because fluid and electrolyte disturbances are common in the elderly, especially in the postoperative period, avoidance of hypotonic fluid administration and monitorization of volume status and electrolytes are crucial.

9.2 Perioperative management for noncardiac surgery in patients with aortic stenosis

Regarding noncardiac operations, postponing elective surgery is recommended for patients with symptomatic severe AS or asymptomatic severe AS in whom evaluation of the valve has not been done within the last year (Fleisher et al., 2009). If AVR is not feasible because of comorbidities or patient refusal, mortality risk of noncardiac surgery is approximately 10% in patients with severe AS (Fleisher et al., 2009). Stratification of cardiac risk for noncardiac surgery reported in the current ACC/AHA guidelines is summarized in Table 2 (Fleisher et al., 2009). In patients with mild or moderate AS, no clear recommendation is present (Bonow et al., 2008). In the asymptomatic patient with severe AS, AVR is indicated if concurrent CABG operation is required; if EF is below 50%; or if likelihood of rapid progression is high (Bonow et al., 2008). If symptoms are equivocal, an exercise test can be performed and AVR may be planned if symptoms or hypotension occur during the test. Beta blocker treatment should be continued if class I indications for it exist. If the patient is not using beta blockers and has CAD or more than one cardiac risk factor, titration of beta blockers to heart rate and blood pressure is recommended if the patient will undergo high- or intermediate-risk surgery (Fleisher et al., 2009). These cardiac risk factors are listed in Table 3. Starting beta blocker treatment in low doses and careful titration is important in elderly patients who are at increased risk for bradycardia and hypotension and thus adverse events like falls. Furthermore, data about the role of beta blockers in intermediate- and low-risk patients and optimal type, dose, timing, duration, and titration of beta blockers are lacking (Fleisher et al., 2009). Withdrawal of beta blockers in the preoperative period is associated with adverse outcomes and should not be done unless necessary. Cessation of metformin and renin angiotensin system blockers, which increase the risk of postoperative lactic acidosis and renal insufficiency respectively, before the surgical procedure is essential. In a recent study by Calleja et al., elderly patients with asymptomatic severe AS had low morbidity rates that were similar to that seen in well-matched patients with mild-to-moderate AS following intermediate-to-low-risk noncardiac surgery (Calleja et al., 2010). No postoperative death or HF was observed until dismissal. However, intraoperative hypotension requiring vasopressor use was more common in patients with asymptomatic severe AS. BNP may also be used to predict postoperative poor outcomes in patients with heart disease undergoing noncardiac surgery, however data about BNP used for this purpose is scarce. Leibowitz et al. suggest that it may be beneficial to measure BNP levels in the preoperative period for this purpose (Leibowitz et al., 2008).

Risk Stratification	Procedure Examples
Vascular (reported CR often more than 5%)	Aortic and other major vascular surgery Peripheral vascular surgery
Intermediate (reported CR generally 1% to 5%)	Intraperitoneal and intrathoracic surgery Carotid endarterectomy Head and neck surgery Orthopedic surgery Prostate surgery
Low (reported CR generally less than 1%)	Endoscopic procedures Superficial procedure Cataract surgery Breast surgery Ambulatory surgery

* Combined incidence of cardiac death and nonfatal myocardial infarction. CR: cardiac risk.

Table 2. Cardiac Risk* Stratification for Noncardiac Surgical Procedures

History of ischemic heart disease
History of compensated or prior heart failure
History of cerebrovascular disease
Diabetes Mellitus
Renal insufficiency (defined as a preoperative serum creatinine of greater than 2 mg/dL).

Table 3. Clinical risk factors for perioperative cardiovascular complications

10. Surgery

Approximately 2% to 5% of elderly individuals aged 75 years present with signs of severe AS and they are scheduled for elective AVR. AVR is the treatment of choice for patients with severe degenerative AS, offering both symptomatic relief and a potential for improved long-term survival (Heinze et al., 2010). The results of the conventional surgery for octogenarians are satisfactory and 5% to 10% of mortality is noted for isolated AVR (Heinze et al., 2010). On the other hand, elderly patients stay longer in the hospitals and intensive care units during the postoperative period (Avery et al., 2001).

In 1912, Theodore Tuffier was the first to attempt opening AS using his finger. Russel Brock and then Bailey used dilatators for stenotic aortic valves. Today more than 1000 patients have aortic valve surgery per year and surgery for AS is more common than it is for aortic insufficiency. (Barbour J.R. & Ikonmidis J.S., 2007). It's obvious that AVR is indicated in all symptomatic patients and asymptomatic patients with severe AS undergoing open heart surgery. The surgery should immediately be programmed if the patient becomes symptomatic. United Kingdom heart valve registry observed 1100 elderly patients (56% women) who underwent AVR and the 30-day mortality was 6.6% (Asimakopoulos, 1997, as cited in Aronow, 2007). The actuarial survival was 89% at 1 year, 79% at 3 years, 69% at 5 years, and 46% at 8 years. The mortality is rising up to 10% per year for the patient who becomes symptomatic. The indications for AVR in patients with AS according to the current ACC/AHA guidelines are listed in Table 4 (Bonow et al., 2006).

Class I
AVR is indicated for symptomatic patients with severe AS.* *(Level of Evidence: B)*
AVR is indicated for patients with severe AS* undergoing coronary artery bypass graft surgery (CABG). *(Level of Evidence: C)*
AVR is indicated for patients with severe AS* undergoing surgery on the aorta or other heart valves. *(Level of Evidence: C)*
AVR is recommended for patients with severe AS* and LV systolic dysfunction (ejection fraction less than 0.50). *(Level of Evidence: C)*
Class IIa
AVR is reasonable for patients with moderate AS* undergoing CABG or surgery on the aorta or other heart valves (see Section 3.7 on combined multiple valve disease and Section 10.4 on AVR in patients undergoing CABG). *(Level of Evidence: B)*
Class IIb
AVR may be considered for asymptomatic patients with severe AS* and abnormal response to exercise (e.g., development of symptoms or asymptomatic hypotension). *(Level of Evidence: C)*
AVR may be considered for adults with severe asymptomatic AS* if there is a high likelihood of rapid progression (age, calcification, and CAD) or if surgery might be delayed at the time of symptom onset. *(Level of Evidence: C)*
AVR may be considered in patients undergoing CABG who have mild AS* when there is evidence, such as moderate to severe valve calcification, that progression may be rapid. *(Level of Evidence: C)*
AVR may be considered for asymptomatic patients with extremely severe AS (aortic valve area less than 0.6 cm^2, mean gradient greater than 60 mm Hg, and jet velocity greater than 5.0 m per second) when the patient's expected operative mortality is 1.0% or less. *(Level of Evidence: C)*
Class III
AVR is not useful for the prevention of sudden death in asymptomatic patients with AS who have none of the findings listed under the class IIa/IIb recommendations. *(Level of Evidence: B)*

Table 4. Indications for Aortic Valve Replacement.

Although the surgery for the asymptomatic patients is preferred due to risk of sudden death, surgery for asymptomatic octogenarians is controversial. The complex cardiac procedures have high risks for elderly patients. The mortality rate of valve surgery and risk of sudden death without surgery have to be carefully considered. Postoperatively symptoms diminish and quality of life is improved in the majority of patients ≥75 years who had undergone aortic valve surgery, but long term survival was not affected (Petersen & Poulsen, 2010).

AVR usually performed under general anesthesia using conventional techniques of open-heart surgery with median sternotomy. Minimally invasive procedures are associated with acceptable mortality and morbidity rates even in high risk patients. Minimally invasive aortic valve surgery can be performed through three different approaches. These are upper mini sternotomy, transverse sternotomy and right parasternal mini thoracotomy, sometimes using port-access technique. This procedure has advantages such as less surgical trauma, decreased pain and faster recovery. Small incisions may also be associated with low infection rates (Olin et al., 1999). It reduces blood transfusions and shortens the length of hospital and ICU stay (Korach et al., 2010). It is a safe operation and is associated with lower incidence of atelectasis in the cardiac ICU (Foghsgaard et al., 2009). Port access aortic surgery also allows patients to be extubated earlier (Wheatley et al., 2004). Avoidance of full sternotomy for osteoporotic elderly patients prompts a comfortable postoperative period.

Although the number of the aortic valve procedures increase worldwide, the ideal valve choice is still a debate. There are several options for valves. These are mechanical valve prostheses, stented and stentless bioprosthetic valves, aortic homografts and pulmonary autografts. The use of these valves differs from patient to patient due to comorbidities and anticoagulant needs. The bioprosthetic valves are good alternatives for elderly patients because long term anticoagulation use is not required.

The other situation for the elderly patients undergoing AVR is the injurious effects of cardiopulmonarybypass to the organs. This results as a systemic inflammatory response and this may influence the post-operative course of the elderly patients adversely.

Paroxysmal or chronic AF and a LVEF <35% is a risk factor for mortality in patients with severe AS undergoing AVR. Of 83 elderly patients with severe AS and an LVEF <35%, 29 (35%) had paroxysmal or chronic AF (Levy, 2006, as cited in Aronow, 2007). The perioperative mortality was 24% in the group with AF versus 5,5% in the group without AF.

11. Transcatheter aortic valve implantation

Surgical AVR is currently the gold-standard treatment for patients with severe symptomatic AS. Without surgery, the prognosis is extremely poor, with a 3-year survival rate of <30%. However, in the huge Euro Heart multinational registry in Europe, 33% of symptomatic patients over the age of 65 years were not referred for surgery. (Iung et al., 2003). The reasons for not planning surgery were not always the co morbidities. David Bach's series showed the same issue and 33% of symptomatic patients were not referred for surgery, some of whom had a low Euro Score risk. (Bach et al., 2007). Balloon aortic valvuloplasty, which was described in the 1980s, was the first alternative to surgical therapy (Cribier et al., 1986). Despite high rates of initial procedural success, restenosis is frequently encountered in the long term. The procedure has generally been abandoned in adult patients except as a palliative procedure often prior to surgical AVR (Eltchaninoff et al., 1995). Trans-catheter aortic valve implantation (TAVI) was first described by Andersen et al in 1992 (Andersen et al., 1992). They implanted an expandable aortic valve by a catheter technique in a closed chest pig model. The first attempt to use TAVI in man was in 2002 by Cribier et al. (Cribier et al., 2002). A percutaneous bioprosthesis was successfully implanted within the diseased native aortic valve through an antegrade transseptal approach. Percutaneous transcatheter implantation of the aortic valve has been utilized as an alternative to open heart surgery in high risk patients with symptomatic severe AS who are not suitable for open surgery. Patients might be considered candidates for TAVI if they fulfill the following criteria: symptomatic severe AS, a life expectancy of >1year, contraindications for surgery, high risk for surgery (clinical judgment plus Euro Score (logistic) >20%; STS Score>10%), and/or porcelain aorta, history of thoracic irradiation, severe thoracic deformity, patent coronary by pass, cachexia, recurrent pulmonary emboli, right ventricular insufficiency and cirrhosis.

Stented valves placed either transapically or percutaneously are garnering much attention (Lichtenstein et al., 2006; Criber et al., 2006). Within these procedures, firstly balloon aortic valvotomy is undertaken and a stented bioprosthesis is then deployed over a balloon into the aortic annulus. Inflation of the balloon anchors the valve in place in the annulus, effectively achieving AVR. Transapical approach necessitates a thoracotomy but the valve is deployed into the beating heart and extracorporeal circulation is not performed. In the percutaneous approach, the valve is deployed either antegradely via the transseptal route, or retrogradely across the native aortic valve. Contraindications for TAVI are as follows: an aortic annulus of <18 mm or >27 mm, bicuspid valves, heavy calcification in front of LM, presence of LV thrombus and need for CABG (relative). Some specific contraindications for transfemoral approach are; narrow peripheral arteries (diameter < 8-9 mm), severe tortuousity or calcification, history of aorto-femoral by pass, aneurysm of abdominal aorta with thrombosis, and severe atheroma of the arch. TAVI has revolutionized the management of patients with severe AS, with more than 10,000 implants performed to date. Two studies corroborated the results of previous reports in a real world population of consecutive patients within their respective countries (Eltchaninoff et al., 2010; Zahn et al., 2011). They demonstrated a technical success rate of 98-99%, similar 30 day mortality rates (12%), and an incidence of stroke of 3-4%. A recently published study (Partner Trial) successfully met both primary and co-primary endpoints with a significant reduction in 1-year mortality (30.7% for TAVI versus 50.7% for standard therapy, p<0.001, Leon et al., 2010). It also demonstrated there was a significant reduction in the composite endpoint of death from any cause or repeat hospitalization (42.5% for TAVI versus 71.6% for standard therapy, p<0.0001). However, TAVI as compared with standard therapy, was associated with a higher incidence of major strokes (5.0% versus 1.1 %, p=0.06) and major vascular complications (16.2% versus 1.1%, p <0.001 Leon et al., 2010). Despite continual technical advancement of TAVI devices and procedures, the combined mortality and morbidity is still high in the range of 5-10%, especially when we are facing a group of high surgical risk patients. In the future when it is a safer and more reliable procedure and further refinement of the device (i.e. smaller size delivery systems and multiple valve size options) is done, utilization of the procedure in patients with lower surgical risk may be possible.

12. Geriatric aspects

12.1 Activities of daily living

Bemmel et al investigated the impact of valvular heart disease on the activities of daily living (ADL, assessed with Groningen Activity Restriction Scale) in eighty one 90-year old individuals (Bemmel et al., 2010). The study population consisted of individuals 78% of whom lived independently and only 35% had history of cardiovascular disease. Most common valve diseases were mitral regurgitation (73%) and aortic regurgitation (47%). AS was present in 17% (14 in 81) of the study population (9 mild, 4 moderate and 1 severe). No correlation between the presence of valve diseases and dependence in ADL was found in this population. It is not feasible to extend these results to the general population because the study population consisted of healthier and cognitively more intact individuals expected for this age. Because significant AS may cause deterioration in ADL via several mechanisms like limitation of functional capacity, depression and cognitive decline due to concomitant atherosclerosis in the central nervous system, studies assessing ADL in individuals with significant AS are needed.

12.2 Frailty

Frailty is a geriatric syndrome which is associated with weakness, instability, limitation, increased vulnerability to stressors, and adverse health outcomes like falls, hospitalization, institutionalization and mortality (Evans et al., 2010). Although there are various definitions to identify individuals with frailty, the most frequently and widely used one was described by Fried and colleagues (Fried et al., 2001; Evans et al., 2010). The following five criteria are used in this definition: poor grip strength, self-reported exhaustion, unexplained weight loss, slow walking speed, and reduced physical activity. An individual having at least three of these criteria is defined as being frail. Patients with significant AS might be prone to become frail. Self-reported exhaustion, slow walking speed and reduced physical activity would be seen in a high percentage of patients with limited physical activity due to exertional dyspnea or angina pectoris associated with significant AS. They may also have weight loss and poor grip strength associated with cardiac cachexia. Assessment of patients with AS about presence of frailty would also be beneficial in perioperative risk assessment as stated in section 9.1. Further studies about the impact of frailty on presence, severity and perioperative risk of AS are needed.

12.3 Malnutrition

Malnutrition is an important health issue in the elderly. Being underweight is associated with more frequent all-cause mortality than being overweight in the elderly (Berrington de Gonzalez et al., 2010). Undernutrition is also associated with tendency to adverse health problems like pressure sores, infections and sarcopenia.

Data assessing the relationship between heart valve problems and malnutrition are very limited. Ikee et al investigated impact of malnutrition-inflammation complex on heart valve calcification in 105 patients on hemodialysis (Ikee et al., 2008). In this study mean age was 67 and aortic (77.4%) and mitral (51.3%) valve calcification rates were very high. They found some association between malnutrition and valve calcification. However, as a marker of malnutrition they used only albumin level which is not specific for malnutrition. Wang et al investigated the association of malnutrition and fetuin-A, which has recently been identified as an important circulating inhibitor of calcification, in 238 patients on peritoneal dialysis treatment (Wang et al., 2005). Nutritional assessment was done with serum albumin levels and subjective global assessment tool in this study. Cardiac valve calcification was present in 26% of the patients. They showed a significant correlation between fetuin-A levels and presence and degree of malnutrition. Otto et al reported increased long-term mortality independently associated with cachexia in 674 elderly patients who underwent balloon aortic valvuloplasty for AS (Otto el al., 1994).

Undernutrition may also influence outcomes after cardiac valve surgery. Tepsuwan et al. assessed the incidence and impact of cardiac cachexia retrospectively in 353 patients who underwent cardiac valve surgery (Tepsuwan et al., 2009). The study population was relatively young and most of them had mitral stenosis or mitral regurgitation. They used the finding of a body weight less than 80% of ideal body weight as cachexia which was present in 13% of the study population. They found significant association between presence of cachexia and worse New York Heart Association functional class, higher incidence of infective endocarditis and tricuspid regurgitation, longer postoperative hospitalization and more frequent postoperative complications and tendency to a higher mortality rate. Thourani et al investigated the impact of body mass index (BMI) on morbidity and mortality

after cardiac valve surgery in 4247 patients (Thourani et al., 2011). Most of their study population underwent isolated AVR (47.2%) or isolated mitral valve procedure (26%). They showed increased in-hospital and all-cause long-term mortality in patients with a BMI of less than 25 compared to patients with a BMI of 25-35 or higher than 35. However they had no laboratory or clinical data about nutritional status. Engelman et al retrospectively assessed impact of BMI and albumin levels on morbidity and mortality after cardiac surgery in 5168 patients undergoing coronary artery bypass or valve operations (Engelman et al., 1999). In their study there was no correlation between albumin levels and BMI. Preoperative low albumin (<2.5 g/dl) and low BMI (<20 kg/m^2) were independently associated with increased postoperative mortality. No nutritional assessment tool was utilized in this study.
Potentially, significant AS may cause malnutrition via different mechanisms. Dietary restriction due to reduced physical capacity and depressive mood may enhance malnutrition. Abdominal angina may also cause avoidance from eating when concomitant systemic atherosclerosis is present in the mesenteric vessels. Further studies specifically investigating the association between malnutrition and AS are needed.

12.4 Depression

Depression is the most common psychiatric disorder in the elderly and later-life depression (LLD) is associated with disability and increased morbidity and mortality (Maixner et al., 2011). Because atypical presentations like somatic symptoms are common and LLD is generally associated with medical comorbidities, recognition is difficult. Study of Bisschop et al., suggested that cardiac disease and arthritis are the most common predisposing factors for medical illness related depression (Bischop et al., 2004). Overall medical illness burden and degree of functional disability may be more important than specific medical illnesses alone (Maixner et al., 2011). Underlying medical illness may affect the prognosis of depression and depression may delay recovery from medical illnesses by decreasing motivation and compliance (Maixner et al., 2011). The importance of screening for depression in patients with heart disease is well established, but identifying patients with depression may be difficult because organic somatic symptoms possibly unrelated to mood may increase the score on depression ratings and many patients with depression deny a depressed mood (Maixner et al., 2011). Nonetheless, many symptoms like insomnia, fatigue, shortness of breath, weight loss, palpitations, and exercise intolerance overlap in heart disease and depression. Even when patients with depression deny sadness, they endorse anhedonia and most other depressive symptoms if further questioning is done (Maixner et al., 2011).

Vascular depression is characterized with late onset or change in course after early onset, persistent symptoms, and association of depression with vascular disease or vascular risk factors and diffuse or multifocal cerebrovascular lesions (Maixner et al., 2011). Although no specific data exist about the association of vascular depression and AS in the elderly, atherosclerosis has pivotal role in the pathogenesis of both conditions.

Among medications possibly precipitating depression are beta blockers, which is being used commonly in patients with heart disease. Although there is conflicting data about the association of beta blockers and depression, and individual susceptibility to depression may be important, patients with risk factors for depression like personal or family history of depression should be followed up in terms of development of depression (Verbeek et al., 2011). Lipophilic beta blockers like propranolol, timolol, pindolol, metoprolol, carvedilol

and nebivolol are more strongly associated with depression than hydrophilic beta blockers like atenolol, nadolol, practolol and sotalol (Verbeek et al., 2011). It is also important not to be reluctant to begin beta blocker treatment when strong indications like CAD exist.
SSRI are widely used in the treatment of depression. There is some data that indicate use of SSRI in patients with CAD and depression may improve cardiovascular outcomes (Kimmel et al., 2011). Because both treatment with SSRI and severe AS may reduce platelet functions, bleeding complications of surgical procedures may be increased in patients with severe AS using SSRI. Because treatment with SSRI may precipitate hyponatremia, monitorization of sodium levels is important in patients using SSRI, especially if older age and concomitant diuretic use is present.

13. Conclusion

Diagnosis and management of AS in the elderly have many differences compared to younger patients. Thus, involvement of experienced staff and utilization of comprehensive assessment in the management of these patients is crucial.

14. References

Ajayi, A.A.; Adigun, A.Q.; Ojofeitimi, E.O.; Yusuph, H. & Ajayi, O.E. (1999). Anthropometric evaluation of cachexia in chronic congestive heart failure: the role of tricuspid regurgitation. *Int J Cardiol*, Vol.71, No.1, (September 1999), pp.79-84.

Ambler, G.; Omar, R.Z.; Royston, P.; Kinsman, R.; Keogh, B.E. & Taylor, K.M. (2005). Generic, simple risk stratification model for heart valve surgery. *Circulation*, Vol.112, No.2, (July 2005), pp.224-31.

Andersen, H.R; Knudsen, L.L; Hasenkam, J.M. (1992). Transluminal implantation of artificial heart valves. Description of a new expandable aortic valve and initial results with implantation by catheter technique in closed chest pigs. *Eur Heart J*. Vol.13, No.5, (May 1992), pp.704-708.

Arnaoutakis, G.J.; George, T.J.; Alejo, D.E.; Merlo, C.A.; Baumgartner, W.A.; Cameron, D.E. & Shah, A.S. (2011). Society of Thoracic Surgeons Risk Score predicts hospital charges and resource use after aortic valve replacement. *J Thorac Cardiovasc Surg*, (15 April 2011). [Epub ahead of print]

Aronow, W.S; Ahn, C; Shirani, J; Kronzon, I. (1998). Comparison of frequency of new coronary events in older persons with mild, moderate, and severe valvular aortic stenosis with those without aortic stenosis. Am J Cardiol. Vol.81, No.5, (March 1998), pp.647- 649.

Aronow, W.S; Kronzon, I. (1991). Prevalence and severity of valvular aortic stenosis determined by Doppler echocardiography and its association with echocardiographic and electrocardiographic left ventricular hypertrophy and physical signs of aortic stenosis in elderly patients. *Am J Cardiol*, Vol. 67, No.8, (March 1991), pp.776–777.

Aronow, W.S. (2007). Valvular aortic stenosis in the elderly. *Cardiol Rev*. Vol.15, No.5, (September, 2007), pp.217-25.

Avery, G.J; Ley, S.J; Hill, J.D; Hershon, J.J & Dick S.E. (2001). Cardiac surgery in the octogenarian: evaluation of risk, cost, and outcome. *Ann Thorac Surg*. Vol.71, No.2, (February, 2001), pp.591-6.

Bach, D.S; Nina, C and Deeb G.M. (2007). Unoperated Patients With Severe Aortic Stenosis. J *Am Coll Cardiol*, Vol.50, No.3, (October 2007), pp. 2018-2019.

Barbour, J.R. & Ikonımidis, J.S. (2007). Aortic Valve Replacement, In: *Johns Hopkins Manual of Cardiothoracic Surgery*, Yuh, DD; Vricella, L.A. & Baumgartner W.A. 561-606. Mc Graw-Hill Companies, ISBN-13:978-0-07-141652-8, United States of America)

Beppu, S; Suzuki, S; Matsuda, H; Ohmori, F; Nagata, S; Miyatake, K. (1993). Rapidity of progression of aortic stenosis in patients with congenital bicuspid aortic valves. *Am J Cardiol*, Vol.71, No.4, (February 1993), pp.322-7.

Bergler-Klein, J.; Klaar, U.; Heger, M.; Rosenhek, R.; Mundigler, G.; Gabriel, H.; Binder, T.; Pacher, R.; Maurer, G. & Baumgartner, H. (2004). Natriuretic peptides predict symptom-free survival and postoperative outcome in severe aortic stenosis. *Circulation*, Vol.109, No.19, (May 2004), pp.2302-8.

Bernstein, L.H.; Zions, M.Y.; Haq, S.A.; Zarich, S.; Rucinski, J.; Seamonds, B.; Berger, S.; Lesley, D.Y.; Fleischman, W. & Heitner, J.F. (2009). Effect of renal function loss on NT-proBNP level variations. *Clin Biochem*, Vol.42, No.10-11, (July 2009), pp.1091-8.

Berrington de Gonzalez, A.; Hartge, P.; Cerhan, J.R.; Flint, A.J.; Hannan, L.; MacInnis, R.J.; Moore, S.C.; Tobias, G.S.; Anton-Culver, H.; Freeman, L.B.; Beeson, W.L.; Clipp, S.L.; English, D.R.; Folsom, A.R.; Freedman, D.M.; Giles, G.; Hakansson, N.; Henderson, K.D.; Hoffman-Bolton, J.; Hoppin, J.A.; Koenig, K.L.; Lee, I.M.; Linet, M.S.; Park, Y.; Pocobelli, G.; Schatzkin, A.; Sesso, H.D.; Weiderpass, E.; Willcox, B.J.; Wolk, A.; Zeleniuch-Jacquotte, A.; Willett, W.C. & Thun, M.J. (2010). Body-mass index and mortality among 1.46 million white adults. *N Engl J Med*, Vol.363, No.23, (December 2010), pp2211-9.

Bhutani, M.S; Gupta, S.C; Markert, R.J; Barde, C.J; Donese, R; Gopalswamy, N. (1995). A prospective controlled evaluation of endoscopic detection of angiodysplasia and its association with aortic valve disease. *Gastrointest Endosc*. Vol.42, No.5, (November 1995), pp.398–402.

Bisschop, M.I.; Kriegsman, D.M.; Deeg, D.J.; Beekman, A.T. & van Tilburg, W. (2004). The longitudinal relation between chronic diseases and depression in older persons in the community: the Longitudinal Aging Study Amsterdam. *J Clin Epidemiol*, Vol.57, No.2, (February 2004), pp.187-94.

Bonow, R.O; Carabello, B.A; Chatterjee, K; de Leon, A.C. Jr.; Faxon, D.P; Freed, M.D; Gaasch W.H, Lytle B.W, Nishimura R.A, O'Gara P.T, O'Rourke R.A, Otto C.M, Shah P.M, Shanewise J.S, Smith S.C. Jr; Jacobs, A.K; Adams, C.D; Anderson J.L; Antman, E.M, Fuster, V; Halperin, J.L; Hiratzka, L.F; Hunt, S.A; Lytle, B.W; Nishimura, R; Page, R.L & Riegel B. (2006). ACC/AHA 2006 practice guidelines for the management of patients with valvular heart disease: Executive Summary. A Report of the American College of Cardiology/ American Heart Association Task Force on Practice Guidelines (Writing Committee to Revise the 1998 Guidelines for the Management of Patients With Valvular Heart Disease). Developed in collaboration with the Society of Cardiovascular Anesthesiologists. Endorsed by the Society for

Cardiovascular Angiography and Interventions and the Society of Thoracic Surgeons. J *Am Coll Cardiol*. Vol.48, No.3, (August, 2006), pp.1-148

Bonow, R.O; Carabello, B.A; Chatterjee, K; de Leon, A.C. Jr.; Faxon, D.P; Freed, M.D; Gaasch W.H, Lytle B.W, Nishimura R.A, O'Gara P.T, O'Rourke R.A, Otto C.M, Shah P.M, Shanewise J.S, Smith S.C Jr, Jacobs, A.K; Adams, C.D; Anderson J.L; Antman, E.M, Fuster, V; Halperin, J.L; Hiratzka, L.F; Hunt, S.A; Lytle, B.W; Nishimura, R; Page, R.L & Riegel B. (2006). ACC/AHA 2006 guidelines for the management of patients with valvular heart disease: a report of the American College of Cardiology/American Heart Association Task Force on Practice Guidelines. *Circulation*. Vol.114, No.5, (August 2006), pp.84–231.

Bonow, R.O.; Carabello, B.A.; Chatterjee, K.; de Leon A.C. Jr.; Faxon, D.P.; Freed, M.D.; Gaasch, W.H.; Lytle, B.W.; Nishimura, R.A.; O'Gara, P.T.; O'Rourke, R.A.; Otto, C.M.; Shah, P.M.; Shanewise, J.S; 2006 Writing Committee Members & American College of Cardiology/American Heart Association Task Force. (2008). 2008 Focused update incorporated into the ACC/AHA 2006 guidelines for the management of patients with valvular heart disease: a report of the American College of Cardiology/American Heart Association Task Force on Practice Guidelines (Writing Committee to Revise the 1998 Guidelines for the Management of Patients With Valvular Heart Disease): endorsed by the Society of Cardiovascular Anesthesiologists, Society for Cardiovascular Angiography and Interventions, and Society of Thoracic Surgeons. *Circulation*, Vol.118, No.15, (October 2008), pp.e523-661.

Bouma, B.J; van Den Brink, R.B; van Der Meulen, J.H; Verheul, H.A; Cheriex, E.C; Hamer, H.P; Dekker, E; Lie, K.I; Tijssen, J.G. (1999). To operate or not elderly pateints with aortic stenosis:the decision and its consequences. *Heart*. Vol.82, No.2, (August 1999), pp.143-8

Braunwald, E. (1990). On the natural history of severe aortic stenosis. *J Am Coll Cardiol*. Vol.15, No.1, (April 1990), pp.1018 -1020.

Calleja, A.M.; Dommaraju, S.; Gaddam, R.; Cha, S.; Khandheria, B.K. & Chaliki, H.P. (2010). Cardiac risk in patients aged >75 years with asymptomatic, severe aortic stenosis undergoing noncardiac surgery. *Am J Cardiol*, Vol.105, No.8, (April 2010), pp.1159-63.

Carabello, B.A. & Paulus, W.J. (2009). Aortic stenosis. Lancet, Vol.373, No.9667, (March 2009), pp. 956-66.

Carabello, B.A & Crawford, M.H. (2003). Aortic stenosis. In: *Crawford* M.H., ed. Current diagnosis and treatment in cardiology, 2nd ed. New York: McGraw-Hill Professional, pp.108-20.

Chambers, J; Bach, D; Dumesnil, J; Otto, C; Shah, P; Thomas, J. (2004). The aortic valve in severe aortic stenosis: No longer acceptable? *J Heart Valve Dis*. Vol.13, No.3, (May 2004), pp.344–346.

Cheng, J.W. & Nayar, M. (2009). A review of heart failure management in the elderly population. *Am J Geriatr Pharmacother*, Vol.7, No.5, (October 2009), pp. 233-49.

Clark, B.A; Shannon, R.P; Rosa, R.M & Epstein, F.H. (1994). Increased susceptibility to thiazide-induced hyponatremia in the elderly. *J Am Soc Nephrol,* Vol.5, No.4, (October 1994), pp. 1106-1111.

Cosmi, J.E; Kort, S; Tunick, P.A; Rosenzweig, B.P; Freedberg, R.S; Katz, E.S; Applebaum, R.M; Kronzon, I. (2002). The risk of the development of aortic stenosis in patients with "benign" aortic valve thickening. *Arch Intern Med,* Vol.162, No.29, (November 2002), pp.2345–2347.

Cowell, S.J; Newby, D.E; Prescott, R.J; Bloomfield, P; Reid, J; Northridge, D.B; Boon, N.A. (2005). A randomized trial of intensive lipid-lowering therapy in calcific aortic stenosis. *N Engl J Med,* Vol.352, No.23, (June 2005), pp. 2389–2397.

Cribier, A; Savin, T; Saoudi, N; Rocha, P; Berland, J; Letac, B. (1986). Percutaneous trans-luminal valvuloplasty of acquired aortic-stenosis in elderly patients alternative to valve-replacement. *Lancet,* Vol.1, No.1, (January 1986), pp.63–7.

Cribier, A; Eltchaninoff, H; Bash, A; Borenstein, N; Tron, C; Bauer, F; Derumeaux, G; Anselme, F; Laborde, F; Leon, M.B. (2002). Percutaneous transcatheter implantation of an aortic valve prosthesis for calcific aortic stenosis: first human case description. *Circulation,* Vol.106, No.24, (December 2002), pp.3006–8.

Cribier, A; Eltchaninoff, H; Tron, C; Bauer, F; Agatiello, C; Nercolini, D; Tapiero, S; Litzler, PY; Bessou, JP; Babaliaros, V. (2006). Treatment of calcific aortic stenosis with the percutaneus heart valve: mid-term follow-up from the initial feasibility studies - the French experience . *J Am Coll Cardiol,* Vol.47, No.6, (March 2006), pp.1214-23.

de Arenaza, D.P.; Pepper, J.; Lees, B.; Rubinstein, F.; Nugara, F.; Roughton, M.; Jasinski, M.; Bazzino, O.; Flather, M. & ASSERT (Aortic Stentless versus Stented valve assessed by Echocardiography Randomised Trial) Investigators. (2010). Preoperative 6-minute walk test adds prognostic information to Euroscore in patients undergoing aortic valve replacement. *Heart,* Vol.96, No.2, (January 2010), pp.113-7.

Eltchaninoff, H.; Cribier, A.; Tron, C.; Anselme, F.; Koning, R.; Soyer, R. & Letac, B. (1995). Balloon aortic valvuloplasty in elderly patients at high-risk for surgery, or inoperable-immediate and mid-term results. Balloon aortic valvuloplasty in elderly patients at high-risk for surgery, or inoperable-immediate and mid-term results. *Eur Heart J,* Vol.16, No.8, (August 1995), pp.1079–84.

Eltchaninoff, H; Prat, A; Gilard, M; Leguerrier, A; Blanchard, D; Fournial, G; Iung, B; Donzeau-Gouge, P; Tribouilloy, C; Debrux, JL; Pavie, A; Gueret, P. (2011). Transcatheter aortic valve implantation: early results of the FRANCE (FRench Aortic National CoreValve and Edwards) registry. *Eur Heart J,* Vol.32, No.2, (January 2011), pp.191–197.

Engelman, D.T.; Adams, D,H.; Byrne, J.G.; Aranki, S.F.; Collins, J.J. Jr.; Couper, G.S.; Allred, E.N.; Cohn, L.H. & Rizzo, R.J. (1999). Impact of body mass index and albumin on morbidity and mortality after cardiac surgery. *J Thorac Cardiovasc Surg,* Vol.118, No.5, (November 1999), pp.866-73.

Evans, W.J.; Paolisso, G.; Abbatecol,a A.M.; Corsonello, A.; Bustacchini, S.; Strollo, F. & Lattanzio, F. (2010). Frailty and muscle metabolism dysregulation in the elderly. *Biogerontology*, Vol.11, No.5, (October 2010), pp.527-36.

Faggiano, P; Aurigemma, G.P; Rusconi, C; Gaasch, W.H. (1996). Progression of valvular AS in adults: literature review and clinical implications. *Am Heart J.* Vol.132, No.2, (August 1996), pp.408–417.

Fleisher, L.A.; Beckman, J.A.; Brown, K.A.; Calkins, H.; Chaikof, E.L.; Fleischmann, K.E.; Freeman, W.K.; Froehlich, J.B.; Kasper, E.K.; Kersten, J.R.; Riegel, B. & Robb, J.F. (2009). 2009 ACCF/AHA focused update on perioperative beta blockade incorporated into the ACC/AHA 2007 guidelines on perioperative cardiovascular evaluation and care for noncardiac surgery: a report of the American college of cardiology foundation/American heart association task force on practice guidelines. *Circulation*, Vol.120, No.21, (November 2009), pp.e169-276.

Foghsgaard, S; Gazi, D; Bach, K; Hansen, H; Schmidt, T.A & Kjaergard, H.K. (2009). Minimally invasive aortic valve replacement reduces atelectasis in cardiac intensive care. *Acute Cardiac Care*, Vol.11, No.3, (September, 2009), pp. 169-72.

Fried, L.P.; Tangen, C.M.; Walston, J.; Newman, A.B.; Hirsch, C.; Gottdiener, J.; Seeman, T.; Tracy, R.; Kop, W.J.; Burke, G. & McBurnie, M.A. (2001). Cardiovascular Health Study Collaborative Research Group. Frailty in older adults: evidence for a phenotype. *J Gerontol A Biol Sci Med Sci*, Vol.56, No.3, (March 2001), pp.M146-56.

Frilling, B.; von Renteln-Kruse, W. & Riess, F.C. (2010). Evaluation of operative risk in elderly patients undergoing aortic valve replacement: the predictive value of operative risk scores. *Cardiology*, Vol.116, No.3, (2010), pp.213-8.

Frogel, J. & Galusca, D. (2010). Anesthetic considerations for patients with advanced valvular heart disease undergoing noncardiac surgery. *Anesthesiol Clin*, Vol.28, No.1, (March 2010), pp.67-85.

Furberg, C.D; Psaty, B.M; Manolio, T.A; Gardin, J.M; Smith, V.E; Rautaharju, P.M. (1994). Prevalence of atrial fibrillation in elderly subjects (The Cardiovascular Health Study). *Am J Cardiol*, Vol.74, No.3, (August 1994), pp.236–241.

Georeeson, S; Mever, K.B; Pauker, S.G. (1990). Decision analysis clinical cardiology: When is coronary angiography required in aortic stenosis. *J Am Coll Cardiol*, Vol.15, No.4, (March 1990), pp.751-62.

Giltay, E.J.; Huijskes, R.V.; Kho, K.H.; Blansjaar, B.A.; Rosseel, P.M. (2006). Psychotic symptoms in patients undergoing coronary artery bypass grafting and heart valve operation. *Eur J Cardiothorac Surg*, Vol.30, No.1, (July 2006), pp.140-7.

Gould, K.L. (1997). Why angina pectoris in aortic stenosis. *Circulation*, Vol.95, No.4, (February 1997), pp.790-2.

Ha, J.W; Lulic, F; Bailey, K.R; Pellikka, P.A; Seward, J.B; Tajik, A.J; Oh, J.K. (2003). Effects of treadmill exercise on mitral inflow and annular velocities in healthy adults. *Am J Cardiol*, Vol.91, No.1, (January 2003), pp.114-5.

Hammermeister, K.; Sethi, G.K.; Henderson, W.G.; Grover, F.L.; Oprian, C. & Rahimtoola, S.H. (2000). Outcomes 15 years after valve replacement with a mechanical versus a bioprosthetic valve: final report of the Veterans Affairs randomized trial. *J Am Coll Cardiol*, Vol.36, No.4, October 2000, pp.1152-8.

Heinze, H; Sier, H; Schäfer, U & Heringlake, M. (2010). Percutaneous aortic valve replacement: overview and suggestions for anesthetic management. *J Clin Anesth*, Vol.22, No.5, (August 2010), pp.373-8.

Hood, W.P Jr; Rackley, C.E; Rolet E.L. (1968). Wall stress in the normal and hypertrophied human left ventricle. *Am J Cardiol*, Vol.22, No.4, (October 1968), pp.550 -558.

Hunt, S.A; Abraham, W.T; Chin, M.H; Feldman, A.M; Francis, G.S; Ganiats, T.G; Jessup, M; Konstam, M.A; Mancini D.M, Michl, K; Oates, J.A; Rahko, P.S; Silver, M.A; Stevenson, L.W; Yancy, C.W. (2009). 2009 focused update incorporated into the ACC/AHA 2005 Guidelines for the Diagnosis and Management of Heart Failure in Adults: a report of the American College of Cardiology Foundation/American Heart Association Task Force on Practice Guidelines: developed in collaboration with the International Society for Heart and Lung Transplantation. *Circulation*, Vol.119, No.14, (April 2009), pp. e391-479.

Hwang, K.S & Kim, G.H. (2010). Thiazide-induced hyponatremia. *Electrolyte Blood Press.* Vol.8, No.1, (June 2010), pp. 51-57.

Ikee, R.; Honda, K.; Oka, M.; Maesato, K.; Mano, T.; Moriya, H.; Ohtake, T. & Kobayashi, S. (2008). Association of heart valve calcification with malnutrition-inflammation complex syndrome, beta-microglobulin, and carotid intima media thickness in patients on hemodialysis. *Ther Apher Dial*, Vol.12, No.6, (December 2008), pp.464-8.

John, A.S; Dill, T; Brandt, R.R; Rau, M; Ricken, W; Bachmann, G; Hamm, C.W. (2003).Magnetic resonance to assess the aortic valve area: How does it compare to current diagnostic standards? *J Am Coll Cardiol*, Vol.42, No.3, (August 2003), pp.519-526.

Johnson, A.M. (1971). Aortic stenosis, sudden death, and the left ventricular baroceptors. *Br Heart J*, Vol.33, No.1, (January 1971), pp.1-5.

Juergens, M.C.; Seekatz, B.; Moosdorf, R.G.; Petrie, K.J. & Rief, W. (2010). Illness beliefs before cardiac surgery predict disability, quality of life, and depression 3 months later. *J Psychosom Res*, Vol.68, No.6, (June 2010), pp.553-60.

Julius, B.K; Spillmann, M; Vassalli, G; Villari, B; Eberli, F.R; Hess, OM. (1997). Angina pectoris in patients with aortic stenosis and normal coronary arteries. Mechanisms and pathophysiological concepts. *Circulation*, Vol.95, No.4, (February 1997). pp.892-8.

Kennedy, J.W; Twiss, R.D; Blackmon, J.R. (1968). Quantitative angiocardiography. III. Relationships of left ventricular pressure, volume and mass in aortic valve disease. *Circulation*, Vol.38, No.5, (November 1968), pp.838–845.

Kimmel, S.E.; Schelleman, H.; Berlin, J.A.; Oslin, D.W.; Weinstein, R.B.; Kinman, J.L.; Sauer, W.H. & Lewis, J.D. (2011). The Effect of Selective Serotonin Reuptake Inhibitors on the Risk of Myocardial Infarction in a Cohort of Patients with Depression. *Br J Clin Pharmacol*, (9 May 2011) [Epub ahead of print].

Korach, A; Shemin, R.J; Hunter, C.T; Bao, Y & Shapira, O.M.(2010). Minimally invasive versus conventional aortic valve replacement: a 10-year experience. *J Cardiovasc Surg (Torino)*, Vol.51, No.3, (June, 2010), pp. 417-21.

Kort, S; Applebaum, R.M; Grossi, E.A; Baumann, G; Colvin, S; Galloway, AC; Ribakove, G.H; Steinberg, B.M; Peada, B; Tunick, P.A & Kronzon, I. (2001). Minimally invasive aortic valve replacement: Echocardiographic and clinical results. *American Heart Journal*, Vol.142, No.3, (September, 2001), pp.476-81.

Leibowitz, D.; Planer, D.; Rott, D.; Elitzur, Y.; Chajek-Shaul, T. & Weiss, AT. (2008). Brain natriuretic peptide levels predict perioperative events in cardiac patients undergoing noncardiac surgery: a prospective study. *Cardiology*, Vol. 110, No.4, (2008), pp.266-70.

Leon, M.B; Smith, C.R; Mack, M; Miller, D.C; Moses, J.W; Svensson, L.G; Tuzcu, E.M; Webb, J.G; Fontana, G.P; Makkar, R.R; Brown, D.L; Block, P.C; Guyton, R.A; Pichard, A.D; Bavaria, J.E; Herrmann, H.C; Douglas, P.S; Petersen, J.L; Akin, J.J; Anderson, W.N; Wang, D; Pocock, S. (2010). Transcatheter Aortic-Valve Implantation for Aortic Stenosis in Patients Who Cannot Undergo Surgery. *N Engl J Med*, Vol.363, No.17, (October 2010), pp.1597-1607.

Levy, D; Garrison, R.J; Savage, D.D; Kannel, W.B; Castelli, W.P. (1990). Prognostic implications of echocardiographically determined left ventricular mass in the Framingham heart study. *N Engl J Med*, Vol.322, No.22, (May 1990), pp.1561–66.

Lichtenstein, S.V; Cheung, A; Ye, J; Thompson, C.R; Carere, R.G; Pasupati, S; Webb, J.G. (2006). Transapical transcathater aortic valve implantation in humans : initial clinical experience . *Circulation*, Vol.114, No. 6, (August 2006), pp.591-96

Licker, M.; Cikirikcioglu, M.; Inan, C.; Cartier, V.; Kalangos, A.; Theologou, T.; Cassina, T. & Diaper, J. (2010). Preoperative diastolic function predicts the onset of left ventricular dysfunction following aortic valve replacement in high-risk patients with aortic stenosis. *Crit Care*, Vol.14, No.3, (2010), p.R101.

Lindroos, M; Kupari, M; Valvanne, J; Strandberg, T; Heikkilä, J; Tilvis, R. (1994). Factors associated with calcific degeneration in the elderly. *Eur Heart J*, Vol15, No.7, (July 1994), pp.865-870.

Lombard, J.T; Selzer, A. (1987). Valvular aortic stenosis. *Ann Intern Med*, Vol.106, No.2, (February 1987), pp.292–298.

Iung, B; Baron, G; Butchart, E.G; Delahaye, F; Gohlke-Bärwolf, C; Levang, O.W; Tornos, P; Vanoverschelde, J.L; Vermeer F, Boersma, E; Ravaud P; Vahanian, A. (2003). A prospective survey of patients with valvular heart disease in Europe: The Euro Heart Survey on valvular heart disease. *Eur Heart J*, Vol. 24, No.13, (July 2003), pp. 1231 - 1243.

Maixner, S.M.; Strubl,e L.; Blazek, M. & Kales, H.C. (2011). Later-life depression and heart failure. *Heart Fail Clin*, Vol.7, No.1, (January 2011), pp.47-58.

Maldonado, J.R.; Wysong, A.; van der Starre, P.J.; Block, T.; Miller, C. & Reitz, B.A. (2009). Dexmedetomidine and the reduction of postoperative delirium after cardiac surgery. *Psychosomatics*, Vol.50, No.3, (May-June 2009), pp.206-17.

Monin, J.L.; Lancellotti, P.; Monchi, M.; Lim, P.; Weiss, E.; Piérard. & Guéret, P. (2009). Risk score for predicting outcome in patients with asymptomatic aortic stenosis. *Circulation,* Vol.120, No.1, (July 2009), pp.69-75.

Monin, J.L.; Quéré, J.P.; Monchi, M.; Petit, H.; Baleynaud, S.; Chauvel, C.; Pop, C.; Ohlmann, P.; Lelguen, C.; Dehant, P.; Tribouilloy, C. & Guéret, P. (2003). Low-gradient aortic stenosis: operative risk stratifi cation and predictors for long-term outcome: a multicenter study using dobutamine stress hemodynamics. *Circulation,* Vol.108, No.3, (July 2003), pp. 319–324.

Moon, D.G; Jin, M.H; Lee, J.G; Kim, J.J; Kim, M.G; Cha, D.R. (2004). Antidiuretic hormone in elderly male patients with severe nocturia: a circadian study. *BJU Int*, Vol.94, No.4, (September 2004), pp.571-575.

Munt, B; Legget, M.E; Kraft, C.D; Miyake-Hull, C.Y; Fujioka, M; Otto, C.M. (1999). Physical examination in valvular aortic stenosis: Correlation with stenosis severity and prediction of clinical outcome. *Am Heart J,* Vol.137, No.2, (February 1999), pp.298-306.

Naqvi, T.Z; Siegel, R.J. (1999). Aortic Stenosis: The Role of Transesophageal Echocardiography. *Echocardiography,* Vol.16, No.7, (October 1999), pp.677–688.

Nashef, S.A.; Roques, F.; Michel, P.; Gauducheau, E.; Lemeshow, S. & Salamon R. (1999). European system for cardiac operative risk evaluation (EuroSCORE). *Eur J Cardiothorac Surg,* Vol.16, No.1, (July 1999), pp. 9-13.

Nkomo, V.T; Gardin, J.M; Skelton, T.N; Gottdiener, J.S; Scott, C.G; Enriquez-Sarano, M. (2006). Burden of valvular heart diseases: a population-based study. *Lancet,* Vol.368, No.9540, (September 2006), pp.1005-11.

Novaro, G.M; Tiong, I.Y; Pearce, G.L; Lauer, M.S; Sprecher, D.L; Griffin, B.P. (2001). Effect of hydroxymethylglutaryl coenzyme a reductase inhibitors on the progression of calcific aortic stenosis. *Circulation,* Vol. 104, No.18, (October 2001), pp. 2205–2209.

Nozohoor, S.; Nilsson, J.; Lührs, C.; Roijer, A.; Algotsson, L. & Sjögren, J. (2009). B-type natriuretic peptide as a predictor of postoperative heart failure after aortic valve replacement. *J Cardiothorac Vasc Anesth,* Vol.23, No.2, (April 2009), pp.161-5.

Olin, C.L & Péterffy, A. (1999). Minimal access aortic valve surgery. *Eur J Cardiothorac Surg,* Vol. 15, No.1, (January, 1999), pp.39-43.

Ortlepp, J.R; Hoffmann, R; Ohme, F; Lauscher J, Bleckmann F, Hanrath P. (2001). The vitamin D receptor genotype predisposes to the development of calcific aortic valve stenosis. *Heart,* Vol.85, No.6, (June 2001), pp.635- 638.

Otto, C.M.; Pearlman, A.S. & Gardner, C.L. (1989). Hemodynamic progression of aortic stenosis in adults assessed by Doppler echocardiography. *J Am Coll Cardiol,* Vol.13, No.3, (March 1989), pp.545–550.

Otto, C.M.; Kuusisto, J.; Reichenbach, D.D.; Gown, A.M. & O'Brien, K.D. (1994). Characterization of the early lesion of 'degenerative' valvular aortic stenosis. *Circulation,* Vol.90, No.2, (August 1994), pp.844–853.

Otto, C.M.; Munt, B.I. & Legget, M.E. (1997). Correlation between physical examination findings and Doppler echocardiography in adults with aortic stenosis. *Circulation*, Vol.96, No.2, (February 1997), pp.157.

Otto C.M, Burwash I.G, Legget M.E, Munt B.I, Fujioka M, Healy N.L, Kraft C.D, Miyake-Hull C.Y, Schwaegler R.G. (1997). Prospective study of asymptomatic valvular aortic stenosis: clinical, echocardiographic, and exercise predictors of outcome. *Circulation*, Vol.95, No.9, (May 1997), pp.2262-2270.

Otto C.M. (1997). Aortic stenosis: echocardiographic evaluation of disease severity, disease progression, and the role of echocardiography in clinical decision making. In *Otto* C.M. (ed): The Practice of Clinical Echocardiography, Philadelphia, W.B. Saunders, 1997.

Otto C.M. (2006). Valvular aortic stenosis: Disease severity and timing of intervention. *J Am Coll Cardiol*, Vol.47, No.11, (June 2006), pp.2141-2151.

Pachulski R.T. & Chan,K.L. (1993). Progression of aortic valve dysfunction in 51 adult patients with congenitalbicuspid aortic valve: assessment and follow up by Doppler echocardiography. *Br Heart J*, Vol.69, No.3, (March 1993), pp.237-40.

Passik, C.S.; Ackermann, D.M.; Pluth, J.R. & Edwards, W.D. (1987). Temporal changes in the causes of aortic stenosis: A surgical pathologic study of 646 cases. *Mayo Clin Proc*, Vol.62, No.2, (February 1987), pp.119-123.

Pedrazzini, G.B.; Masson, S.; Latini, R.; Klersy, C.; Rossi, M.G.; Pasotti, E.; Faletra, F.F.; Siclari, F.; Minervini, F.; Moccetti, T. & Auricchio, A. (2008). Comparison of brain natriuretic peptide plasma levels versus logistic EuroSCORE in predicting in-hospital and late postoperative mortality in patients undergoing aortic valve replacement for symptomatic aortic stenosis. *Am J Cardiol*, Vol.102, No.6, (September 2008), pp.749-54.

Peltier, M.; Trojette, F.; Sarano, M.E.; Grigioni, F.; Slama, M.A. & Tribouilloy, C.M. (2003). Relation between cardiovascular risk factors and nonrheumatic severe calcific aortic stenosis among patients with a three-cuspid aortic valve. *Am J Cardiol*, Vol.91, No.1, (January 2003), pp.97-99.

Petersen R.S & Poulsen A. (2010). Quality of life after aortic valve-replacement in patients > or = 75 years. *Ugeskr Laeger*, Vol.172, No.5, (February, 2010), pp.355-9.

Pohle, K.; Dimmler, A.; Feyerer, R.; Feger, S.; Ropers, D.; Daniel, W.G. & Achenbach, S. (2004). Quantification of aortic valve calcification with electron beam tomography: a histomorphometric validation study. *Invest Radiol*, Vol.39, No.4, (April 2004), pp.230-234.

Rajamannan, N.M; Otto, C.M. (2004) Targeted therapy to prevent progression of calcific aortic stenosis. *Circulation*, Vol.110, No.10, (September 2004), pp.1180-1182.

Richards, A.M; Nicholls, M.G; Ikram, H. (1984). Syncope in aortic valvular stenosis. *Lancet*, Vol.17, No.2, (November 1984), pp.1113-6.

Rodés-Cabau, J.; Webb, J.G.; Cheung, A.; Ye, J.; Dumont, E.; Feindel, C.M.; Osten, M.; Natarajan, M.K.; Velianou, J.L.; Martucci, G.; DeVarennes, B.; Chisholm, R.; Peterson, M.D.; Lichtenstein, S.V.; Nietlispach, F.; Doyle, D.; DeLarochellière, R.; Teoh, K.; Chu, V.; Dancea, A.; Lachapelle, K.; Cheema, A.; Latter, D. & Horlick, E.

(2010). Transcatheter aortic valve implantation for the treatment of severe symptomatic aortic stenosis in patients at very high or prohibitive surgical risk: acute and late outcomes of the multicenter Canadian experience. *J Am Coll Cardiol*, Vol.55, No.11, (March 2010), pp.1080-1090.

Rosenhek, R.; Binder, T.; Porenta, G.; Lang, I.; Christ, G.; Schemper, M.; Maurer, G. & Baumgartner, H. (2000). Predictors of outcome in severe, asymptomatic aortic stenosis. *N Engl J Med*, Vol.343, No.9, (May 2000), pp.611- 617.

Rosenhek, R.; Rader, F.; Loho, N.; Gabriel, H.; Heger, M.; Klaar, U.; Schemper, M.; Binder, T.; Maurer, G. & Baumgartner, H. (2004). Statins but not angiotensin-converting enzyme inhibitors delay progression of aortic stenosis. *Circulation*, Vol.110, No.10, (September 2004), pp.1291-1295.

Rosenhek, R.; Iung, B.; Tornos, P.; Antunes, M.J.; Prendergast, B.D.; Otto, C.M.; Kappetein, A.P.; Stepinska, J.; Kaden, J.J.; Naber, C.K.; Acartürk, E. & Gohlke-Bärwolf, C. (2011). ESC Working Group on Valvular Heart Disease Position Paper: assessing the risk of interventions in patients with valvular heart disease. *Eur Heart J*, 2011 Mar 15. [Epub ahead of print]

Ross Jr., J. & Braunwald, E. (1968). Aortic stenosis. *Circulation*, Vol.38, No.1, (April 1968), pp.61-67.

Rossebø, A.B; Pedersen, T.R; Boman, K; Brudi, P; Chambers, J.B; Egstrup, K; Gerdts, E; Gohlke-Bärwolf, C; Holme, I; Kesäniemi, Y.A; Malbecq, W; Nienaber, C.A; Ray, S; Skjaerpe, T; Wachtell, K; Willenheimer, R. (2008). Intensive lipid lowering with simvastatin and ezetimibe in aortic stenosis. *N Engl J Med*, Vol.359, No.13, (September 2008), pp.1343-1356.

Sciomer, S.; Badagliacca, R.; Vizza, C.D. & Fedele, F. (2004). Echocardiography in aortic stenosis: New insights into challenging scenarios. *Ital Heart J*, Vol.5, No.6, (June 2004), pp.457-465.

Steinlechner, B.; Zeidler, P.; Base, E.; Birkenberg, B.; Ankersmit, H.J.; Spannagl, M.; Quehenberger, P.; Hiesmayr, M. & Jilma B. (2011). Patients with severe aortic valve stenosis and impaired platelet function benefit from preoperative desmopressin infusion. *Ann Thorac Surg*, Vol.91, No.5, (May 2011), pp.1420-6.

Stewart, B.F; Siscovick, D; Lind, B.K; Gardin, J.M; Gottdiener, J.S; Smith, V.E; Kitzman, D.W; Otto, C.M. (1997). Clinical factors associated with calcific aortic valve disease. *J Am Coll Cardiol*, Vol.29, No.23, (March 1997), pp.630-634.

Suojaranta-Ylinen, R.T.; Soisalon-Soinine,n S.; Kaartinen, M.; Maasilta, P.K.; Vainikka, T.L.; Vento, A.E. & Salminen, U.S. (2009). Outcome of aortic valve replacement with bioprostheses in the elderly. *J Heart Valve Dis*, Vol.18, No.5, (September 2009), pp.514-23.

Sündermann, S.; Dademasch, A.; Praetorius, J.; Kempfert, J.; Dewey, T.; Falk, V.; Mohr, F.W. & Walther, T. (2011). Comprehensive assessment of frailty for elderly high-risk patients undergoing cardiac surgery. *Eur J Cardiothorac Surg*, Vol.39, No.1, (January 2011), pp.33-7.

Tagore, R.; Ling, L.H.; Yang, H.; Daw, H.Y.; Chan, Y.H. & Sethi, S.K. (2008). Natriuretic peptides in chronic kidney disease. *Clin J Am Soc Nephrol*, Vol.3, No.6, (November 2008), pp.1644-51.

Tepsuwan, T.; Schuarattanapong, S.; Woragidpoonpol, S.; Kulthawong, S.; Chaiyasri, A. & Nawarawong, W. (2009). Incidence and impact of cardiac cachexia in valvular surgery. *Asian Cardiovasc Thorac Ann*, Vol.17, No.6, (December 2009), pp.617-21.

Thourani, V.H.; Keeling, W.B.; Kilgo, P.D.; Puskas, J.D.; Lattouf, O.M.; Chen, E.P. & Guyton, R.A. (2011). The impact of body mass index on morbidity and short- and long-term mortality in cardiac valvular surgery. *J Thorac Cardiovasc Surg*, (28 March 2011). [Epub ahead of print]

Tunick, P.A; Rosenzweig, B.P; Katz, E.S; Freedberg, R.S; Perez, J.L; Kronzon, I. (1994). High risk for vascular events in patients with protruding aortic atheromas: A prospective study. *J Am Coll Cardiol*, Vol.23, No.5, (April 1994 , pp.1085–1090.

Vahanian, A.; Baumgartner, H.; Bax, J.; Butchart, E.; Dion, R.; Filippatos, G.; Flachskampf, F.; Hall, R.; Iung, B.; Kasprzak, J.; Nataf, P.; Tornos, P.; Torracca, L.; Wenink, A; Task Force on the Management of Valvular Hearth Disease of the European Society of Cardiology & ESC Committee for Practice Guidelines. (2007). Guidelines on the management of valvular heart disease: The Task Force on the Management of Valvular Heart Disease of the European Society of Cardiology. *Eur Heart J*, Vol.28, No.2, (January 2007), pp.230-68.

van Bemmel, T.; Delgado, V.; Bax, J.J.; Gussekloo, J.; Blauw, G.J.; Westendorp, R.G. & Holman, E.R. (2010). Impact of valvular heart disease on activities of daily living of nonagenarians: the Leiden 85-plus study a population based study. *BMC Geriatr*,. Vol.10, (April 2010), p.17.

Vengala, S.; Nanda, N.C.; Dod, H.S.; Singh, V., Agrawal, G.; Sinha, A.; Khanna, D.; Upendram, S.K.; Chockalingam, A.; McGiffin, D.C.; Kirklin, J.K. & Pacifico, A.D. (2004). Images in geriatric cardiology. Usefulness of live three-dimensional transthoracic echocardiography in aortic valve stenosis evaluation. *Am J Geriatr Cardiol*, Vol.13, No.5, (September 2004), pp.279–284.

Verbeek, D.E.; van Riezen, J.; de Boer, R.A.; van Melle, J.P. & de Jong P. (2011). A review on the putative association between beta-blockers and depression. *Heart Fail Clin*, Vol.7, No.1, (January 2011), pp.89-99.

Villari, B; Hess, O.M; Kaufmann, P; Krogmann, O.N; Grimm, J; Krayenbuehl, H.P. (1992). Effect of aortic valve stenosis (pressure overload) and regurgitation (volume overload) on left ventricular systolic and diastolic function. *Am J Cardiol*, Vol.69, No.9, (April 1992), pp.927-34.

Wang, A.Y.; Woo, J.; Lam, C.W.; Wang, M.; Chan, I.H.; Gao, P.; Lui, S.F.; Li, P.K. & Sanderson, J.E. (2005). Associations of serum fetuin-A with malnutrition, inflammation, atherosclerosis and valvular calcification syndrome and outcome in peritoneal dialysis patients. *Nephrol Dial Transplant*, Vol.20, No.8, (August 2005), pp.1676-85.

Weidemann, F.; Herrmann, S.; Störk, S.; Niemann, M.; Frantz, S.; Lange, V.; Beer, M.; Gattenlöhner, S.; Voelker, W.; Ertl, G. & Strotmann, J.M. (2009) Impact of myocardial fibrosis in patients with symptomatic severe aortic stenosis. *Circulation*, Vol.120, No.7, (August 2009), pp.577-84.

Wheatley, G.H; Prince, S.L; Herbert, M.A & Ryan, W.H. (2004). Port-access aortic valve surgery: a technique in evolution. *Heart Surg Forum*, Vol.7, No.6, (January, 2004), pp.628-31.

Zahn, R; Gerckens, U; Grube, E; Linke, A; Sievert, H; Eggebrecht, H; Hambrecht, R; Sack, S; Hauptmann, K.E; Richardt G; Figulla, H.R; Senges, J. (2011). Transcatheter aortic valve implantation: first results from a multi-centre real-world registry. *Eur Heart J*, Vol.32, No.2, (January 2011), pp.198–204.

Zile, M.R; Brutsaert, D.L. (2002). New concepts in diastolic dysfunction and diastolic heart failure: part II—causal mechanisms and treatment. *Circulation*, Vol .105, No.12, (Mach 2002), pp.1503–08.

3

Anaesthetic Considerations for Patients with Severe Aortic Stenosis

Subhamay Ghosh, Lajos Bogar and Ahmed Sabry
Department of Anaesthesiology and Intensive Care, University of Pecs, Pecs, Hungary

1. Introduction

Valvular heart disease has significant effect on the outcome of practically any kind of surgical procedure involving general or regional anaesthesia. The most frequently encountered cardiac valve lesions produce pressure overload (mitral stenosis, aortic stenosis) or volume load (mitral regurgitation, aortic regurgitation) on the left atrium or left ventricle. Anaesthetic management during the perioperative period is based on the likely effects of drug induced changes in cardiac rhythm, heart rate, preload, afterload, myocardial contractility, systemic blood pressure, systemic vascular resistance and pulmonary vascular resistance relative to the pathophysiology of the heart disease.[1]

1.1 Clinical essentials of aortic valve disease

Timely diagnosis and treatment of diseases of the aortic valve is essential to avoid fatalities such as intra or post-operative heart failure, severe infection, in extreme cases sepsis, or even sudden death. Some patients present with severe symptoms, whereas others have few or hardly any symptoms at all. The diagnosis may be made on a routine physical examination performed at the ward or a pre-operative assessment. Regular medical follow-up, treatment to prevent infection of the valve (infective endocarditis), and optimal timing of surgery are necessary to avoid the severe consequences of improper functioning of the aortic valve. [2]

As described earlier the ability of the left ventricle to generate the stroke volume (SV) depends on adequate filling or "preload," the contractile state of the muscle, and the impedance to ejection ("afterload"). Valvular lesions impose additional requirements for compensation. Thus, stenotic lesions require the heart to force an adequate volume through a small orifice; regurgitant lesions on the other hand require the heart to eject a large volume because part of the ejected volume returns backwards. Compensation involves both the myocardium and the peripheral vasculature. Preoperative assessment in all patients with valve disease should include a recent (i.e. at least within 6 months) evaluation such as echocardiography, and a detailed assessment of symptom progression [3].

It is very important to Assess, Plan and Administer.

Asses the degree of the valvular lesion preoperatively

Plan with a multidisciplinary team based on the assessment

Administer the proposed drug therapy particularly antibiotics.

The severity and extent of aortic stenosis is of great value for risk assessment and for the design of a therapeutic plan. The plan which involves a detailed preoperative assessment and preparation, intra-operative caution and strict monitoring and post operative care can be further complicated with the association of other anomalies like genetic disorders, auto immune disorders or severe obesity.

2. How valvular disease affects anaesthetic procedures

Aortic stenosis is the commonest of the major valve lesions. While rheumatic disease was historically the most important cause, this has been displaced by degeneration of congenital bicuspid disease. This latter abnormality occurs in 1-2% of the population. Elderly patients may also have significant "senile" degeneration of a normal (tricuspid) aortic valve. Both rheumatic disease and congenital bicuspid disease become hemodynamically significant over a period of decades, with patients presenting with symptoms and the need for valve replacement usually during or after the 5th decade.[3] The gradual process of narrowing of the aortic orifice leads to concentric left ventricular hypertrophy and a reduction in left ventricular compliance - the myocardium becomes thick, the end-diastolic pressure rises, but there is no dilatation. Typically this occurs as the valve area decreases over years from the normal 2.5 - 3.5 cm^2 to about 1 cm^2. The left ventricle generates very high systolic pressures to overcome the stenosis, but aortic pressures are normal. Because of the decreased compliance, LV filling during diastole depends on adequate preload as well as atrial contraction. While the latter contributes less than 20% of filling in the normal heart, it may contribute twice this amount in AS. This phase of AS is termed "mild" stenosis with physiologic compensation. As the aortic valve area diminishes below 1 cm^2 down to 0.5 cm^2, the stenosis is termed "moderate." Patients begin to develop symptoms as the heart struggles to maintain flow through the narrowing lesion. The increased work of the heart in association with decreased compliance and increased LVEDP results in angina in the majority of patients. This occurs in the absence of coronary artery disease (CAD), although up to 50% of patients may have significant CAD.[4] The left ventricle begins to dilate, the atrium may develop fibrillation, and the patient begins to experience symptoms of pulmonary congestion or even syncope with any type of excitement or exertion. "Critical" stenosis is present if the valve area is less than 0.5 cm^2. The onset of angina is associated with an average survival of 5 years; heart failure or syncope are associated with less than 3 years survival.[5] Valve replacement is recommended when the valve area is less than 0.8 cm^2 or if there is ventricular dysfunction, ventricular ectopy or an inadequate blood pressure response to exercise. Percutaneous balloon valvuloplasty is possible in selected patients.

2.1 The detailed assessment

2.1.1 Preoperative assessment

The main aim of such an assessment is to determine the risks of the patient suffering from peri and/or postoperative deterioration of health and plan its prevention. Severe valvular disease in patients presenting for noncardiac surgery is a major predictor of increased peri-operative cardiovascular risk, mandating intensive management that may result in delay or cancellation of, or pre-operative intervention before, surgery except in the case of emergency surgery[4]. Symptomatic stenotic lesions (aortic and mitral valve stenosis) are associated with a higher risk of peri-operative cardiac complications than symptomatic regurgitation (aortic or mitral valve insufficiency), which is usually better tolerated in the peri-operative setting or may even be stabilized pre-operatively with medical pretreatment[4]. The valvular disease with the highest risk for the non-cardiac surgical patient is severe aortic stenosis.

2.1.1.1 Meeting the patient

A review of the patient's history and medical records to be sure the degree of stenosis, both clinically and objectively is appreciated. This review may result in a referral for valve replacement or valvuloplasty. Questions designed to define exercise tolerance are necessary to evaluate cardiac reserve to provide a functional classification according to the criteria established by the New York Heart Association (NYHA). When myocardial contractility is impaired patients complain of dyspnoea, orthopnea, and easy fatigability, a compensatory increase in the sympathetic nervous system activity may manifest as anxiety, diaphoresis, and resting tachycardia. Congestive heart failure (CHF) is a frequent complication of chronic valvular heart disease and its presence is noted by basilar chest rales, jugular venous distension and a third heart sound on physical examination. Cardiac dysrhythmias are common with valvular heart disease; angina pectoris may occur in patients with valvular heart disease even in the absence of coronary disease due to increased myocardial oxygen consumption and demand for the hypertrophied myocardium. Valvular heart disease and ischemic heart disease (IHD) frequently co-exist. 50% of patients with aortic stenosis who are older than 50 year of age have associated IHD. The presence of CAD with mitral or aortic valve disease worsens the long term prognosis.

Class	Description
I	Asymptomatic
II	Symptoms with ordinary activity but comfortably at rest
III	Symptoms with minimal activity but comfortable at rest
IV	symptoms at rest

Table 1. NYHA functional classification of patients with heart disease [1]

2.1.1.2 Charting out the assessment form

Filling out the assessment form is the very backbone of the procedure to follow. Apart from the neurological, cardiac, respiratory, nephrology, gastrointestinal history, it is very important to discuss the use of the patient's own medication prior to the surgical procedure. Allergies and complications during previous procedures should not be neglected. Detailed information should be availed regarding the discontinuation of anticoagulants like clopidogrel and its substitution by low molecular weight heparin 10 days before and immediately after the procedure.

2.1.1.3 Discussing anaesthesia with the patient

The patient should be informed about the procedure preferably in the presence of the surgeon. This way any question regarding the surgical details of the procedure can be answered appropriately. The patient has to be informed clearly regarding the steps of the anaesthetic procedure starting from leaving the ward through the events in the operating theatre until reaching the intensive care unit. He/she needs to be reassured about optimal analgesia during the procedures involved. Proper information regarding the risks of the anaesthetic procedure and their possible solutions should be clarified.

2.1.1.4 Discussing the procedure with the relative, *parent in case of child*

In many cases patients prefer the preoperative assessment in the presence of their spouse or a relative. In case of children informed consent from the parent is essential. Any major surgical procedure and particularly cardiac surgery may spark fear of death during the procedure amongst patients and their relatives. Questions like 'Will I wake up after the procedure?' should be answered correctly, reassuring the patient and their relatives about the safety of the anaesthetic equipment, skill and care. Informed consent is essential prior to emergency procedures as well.

2.1.1.5 Discussing the anaesthetic plan with the surgical/interdisciplinary team

Details regarding the anaesthetic procedure and postoperative care need to be discussed well with the surgical side for each patient in order for allowing swift coordination and reduction of the possibility of error. In many cases not just the surgeon and the anaesthesiologist is involved but suggestions, investigations, examinations and consultation is required form cardiologists, obstetricians, psychiatrists, neurologists or other specialists. It is therefore essential to form a multidisciplinary team to ensure safe practice. The use of multidisciplinary protocols and drills are advised for emergency procedures.

2.1.1.6 Preparing the patient for surgery

The preparations start from the point the patient has been assessed pre-operatively but prior to the procedure it is essential that the anaesthetist personally visits the patient and preferably accompanies her or him to the operation theatre. Anxiety can cause serious problems before surgery. Anxiolysis might decrease the patient's anxiety and hence decrease the sympathetic output which increases the heart rate, an undesirable parameter in patients with aortic stenosis, digitalis, ß blockers can be used for heart rate control which is essential for ventricular filling. Therefore pre-medication and anxiolytics hold an important place in preparing the patient for surgery. Introduction to the staff in theatre and friendly behaviour creates a stress free environment are useful to avoid unnecessary cardiovascular complications.

Pre-operative management depends on the urgency of surgery and includes the following options:

- open surgical repair before the non-cardiac surgical procedure;
- balloon valvuloplasty before the non-cardiac surgical procedure;
- clearance for surgery without further pre-operative intervention;
- cancellation.

In recently published guidelines[6], it is recommended that, if the aortic stenosis is severe and symptomatic, elective non-cardiac surgery should be postponed and aortic valve replacement performed before elective surgery. If the patient is not a candidate for valve replacement or surgery is semi-elective, balloon valvuloplasty may be performed.

In patients without left ventricular failure, the mortality following aortic valve replacement ranges from 2% to 9% in most centres and may be as low as 1% in patients under the age of 70 years. Concomitant coronary artery disease and poor left ventricular (LV) function are the most important variables affecting overall survival rate [7, 8].

If the patients are not candidates for aortic valve replacement or balloon valvuloplasty, non-cardiac surgery may be performed without pre-operative intervention in a selected group of patients at an acceptably low risk, probably because peri-operative anaesthesiological and surgical management has improved substantially over the past decade[9, 10]. In two recent studies, peri-operative mortality ranged from 1.9% to 7.1%. Peri-operative morbidity included pulmonary oedema in 17.3% of cases, which was effectively treated, and myocardial infarction in 1.9%[9, 10].

2.1.1.6.1 Premedication

Anxiolysis might decease the patient's anxiety and hence decrease the sympathetic output which increases the heart rate, an undesirable parameter in patients with aortic stenosis, digitalis, ß blockers can be used for heart rate control which is essential for ventricular filling.[1]
Introduction to the staff in theatre and friendly behaviour creates a stress free environment are useful to avoid unnecessary cardiovascular complications.

2.1.1.6.2 Endocarditis prophylaxis

Prophylaxis against infective endocarditis is reasonable for the following patients at highest risk for adverse outcomes from infective endocarditis who undergo dental procedures that involve manipulation of either gingival tissue or the periapical region of teeth or perforation of the oral mucosa[11]:

- Patients with prosthetic cardiac valve or prosthetic material used for cardiac valve repair.
- Patients with previous infective endocarditis.
- Patients with CHD.
- Unrepaired cyanotic CHD, including palliative shunts and conduits.
- Completely repaired congenital heart defect repaired with prosthetic material or device, whether placed by surgery or by catheter intervention, during the first 6 months after the procedure.
- Repaired CHD with residual defects at the site or adjacent to the site of a prosthetic patch or prosthetic device (both of which inhibit endothelialization).
- Cardiac transplant recipients with valve regurgitation due to a structurally abnormal valve.

Prophylaxis against infective endocarditis is not recommended for nondental procedures (such as transoesophageal echocardiogram, esophagogastroduodenoscopy, or colonoscopy) in the absence of active infection. *[11]*

2.2 Monitoring during anaesthesia

2.2.1 Non-invasive monitoring

2.2.1.1 ECG

Although even a single post-operative ECG demonstrating ischemia in the recovery room is predictive of a major cardiac complication later during the hospital stay, ECG monitoring alone is not adequate to detect ischemia in real time in the intensive care unit (ICU) and intraoperative settings [12-14]. Specifically, conventional visual ECG monitoring for the detection of transient ST segment changes is inaccurate[14]. Although lead V5 has been known as the best choice for the detection of intraoperative ischemia for many years [15, 16] one study found that lead V4 was more sensitive and appropriate than lead V5 for detecting prolonged post-operative ischemia and infarction [17]. Leads are not specific for ischemic events, and, furthermore, ischemic events are dynamic and may not always appear in the same lead. If a single lead is used for monitoring, there is an increased risk of missing ischemic events. With the use of selected lead combinations, more ischemic events can be precisely diagnosed in the intraoperative setting. In one study, although the best sensitivity was obtained with lead V5 (75%), followed by lead V4 (61%), combining leads V4 and V5 increased the sensitivity to 90%.198 In the same study, when three leads (II, V4, and V5) were used simultaneously, the sensitivity increased to 96%.198 Similarly, in another study in which two or more precordial leads were used, the sensitivity of ECG monitoring was >95% for detection of perioperative ischemia and infarction [17]. It was also shown that ECG monitoring with fewer leads (as few as three leads) had lower sensitivity than monitoring with 12 leads, and there was a statistically significant association, independent of perioperative troponin values, between perioperative ischemia on a 12-lead ECG and long-term mortality [18-20]. Thus, 12-lead ECG monitoring is recommended especially with high-risk patients.

	Agent	Adult**	Children**
Oral	Amoxicillin	2 g	50 mg/kg
Unable to take oral medication	Ampicillin Cefazolin or ceftriaxone	2 g IM or IV 1 g IM or IV	50 mg/kg IM or IV 50 mg/kg IM or IV
Allergic to penicillins or ampicillin—oral	Cephalexin†‡ Clindamycin Azithromycin or clarithromycin	2 g 600 mg 500 mg	50 mg/kg 20 mg/kg 15 mg/kg
Allergic to penicillins or ampicillin and unable to take oral medication	Cefazolin or ceftriaxone‡ Clindamycin	1 g IM or IV 600 mg IM or IV	50 mg/kg IM or IV 20 mg/kg IM or IV

†Or use other first- or second-generation oral cephalosporin in equivalent adult or pediatric dosage.
‡Cephalosporins should not be used in an individual with a history of anaphylaxis, angioedema, or urticaria with penicillins or ampicillin.
IM indicates intramuscular; and IV, intravenous.
** Regimen single dose 30-60 min before the procedures.

Table 2. Regimens for dental procedures

Recommendation	**Class[a]**	**Level[b]**
12-lead ECG monitoring is recommended for all patients undergoing surgery	I	C
Selected lead combinations for better ischemia detection in operation room should be considered	II_a	B

ECG, electrocardiograph. [a] Class of recommendation. [b] Level of evidence.

Table 3. Recommendations on 12-lead ECG monitoring

2.2.1.1.1 Other routine non-invasive monitoring

Standard non-invasive procedures also apply including pulse oximetry, end tidal carbon dioxide monitoring with capnograph, and temperature measurement.

2.2.2 Invasive haemodynamic monitoring

2.2.2.1 Transoesophageal echocardiography

TOE is recommended if acute and severe haemodynamic instability or life-threatening abnormalities develop during or after surgery[21].The main advantage of TOE over pulmonary artery catheterization is the more comprehensive evaluation of cardiac structure and function. Information is quickly available on regional or global, right and/or LV dysfunction, the presence of tamponade or cardiac thrombi, and preload estimation through the measurement of end-diastolic volume. Numerous indices of ventricular and atrial function have been proposed. However, most parameters are load dependent. The role of TOE for haemodynamic monitoring in patients at risk is more controversial. Automated analysis systems exist but are not yet sufficiently validated. There is no evidence that haemodynamic monitoring by TOE accurately stratifies risk or predicts outcome. TOE can be useful in the operating room in patients with severe valvular lesions. The loading conditions during general anaesthesia differ from those present in the preoperative evaluation. Functional and ischemic mitral regurgitation are usually reduced during general anaesthesia. Organic mitral regurgitation can, conversely, increase. In the setting of severe mitral regurgitation, the LV ejection fraction overestimates LV function, and other parameters may be more accurate, such as myocardial velocities or deformation obtained by tissue Doppler imaging or 2D speckle tracking, an angle independent method. These are promising techniques, but more validation is needed before they can be used routinely in this setting. In patients with severe aortic stenosis, appropriate preload is important during surgery. Monitoring of LV end-diastolic volume may be more accurate than that of pulmonary capillary pressure. An appropriate heart rate is crucial in patients with mitral stenosis and aortic regurgitation: a long diastolic period in the former and shorter duration of diastole in the latter. When inappropriate control of heart rate occurs, the consequences should be assessed: changes in transmitral mean gradient and pulmonary arterial pressures in mitral stenosis and changes in LV volumes and indices of LV function in aortic regurgitation.

Recommendations on intraoperative and/or perioperative TOE in patients with or at risk of haemodynamic instability	**Class[a]**	**Level[b]**
TOE is recommended when acute sustained severe haemodynamic disturbances develop during surgery or in the perioperative period	I	C
TOE monitoring may be considered in patients at increased risk of significant haemodynamic disturbances during and after major non-cardiac surgery	II$_b$	C
TOE monitoring may be considered in patients who present severe valvular lesions during major non-cardiac surgical procedures accompanied by significant haemodynamic stresses	II$_b$	C

TOE, transoesophageal echocardiography. [a] Class of recommendation. [b] Level of evidence.

2.2.2.2 Invasive arterial blood pressure monitoring

Invasive arterial blood pressure (IABP) measurement by means of an intra-arterial cannula is a key monitoring technique in high-risk patients both intra-operatively and on the intensive care or high-dependency unit. In addition to giving beat-to-beat blood pressure, the IABP system is increasingly being utilized as the basis of a variety of real-time haemodynamic monitoring systems based on pulse pressure1 or contour.[22]
Its use in Aortic stenosis setting will allow real time beat to beat visualization and hence being proactive rather than reactive to any changes in blood pressure a parameter whose narrow fluctuations might decompromise the haemodynamics in tight valve lesions.

2.2.2.3 The pulmonary artery catheter

Aortic stenosis subjects the left ventricle to excessive afterload, resulting in hypertrophy and a loss of compliance. Unlike the afterload imposed by hypertension, the systemic circulation and especially the coronary circulation are subjected to reduced rather than elevated pressures. Coronary blood flow is impaired by systemic afterload reduction, increased ventricular diastolic pressure and tachycardia which reduces diastolic perfusion time, all may result in angina. Preload must be maintained for the left ventricle to generate an adequate cardiac output across the stenotic valve. Given a noncompliant ventricle, small changes in fluid loading result in large changes in filling pressures.
Critical aortic stenosis creates a narrow window of appropriate fluid loading. Small decrease in preload due to haemorrhage or regional anaesthesia may result in decreased cardiac output and clinical hypotension. Small increases in vascular volume may cause dramatic increases in filling pressures, resulting in pulmonary oedema.
The goal of haemodynamic management should be to maintain filling pressures within the narrow therapeutic window and to avoid tachycardia.***[23]***

2.2.2.4 Glucose monitoring

Diabetes mellitus is an important risk factor for perioperative cardiac complications and death. This condition promotes atherosclerosis, endothelial dysfunction, and activation of platelets and proinflammatory cytokines. Surgical stress is associated with haemodynamic stress and vasospasm and further enhances the prothrombotic state, while inhibiting fibrinolysis. Hyperglycaemia in the absence of established diabetes plays an important role, emphasizing the need for pre-operative management of hyperglycaemia where possible.
Importantly, impaired glucose tolerance is often identified only after glucose loading. Data from the International Diabetes Foundation reveal a high and increasing prevalence of diabetes in Europe, rising from 7.8% in 2003 to 8.4% in 2007, with an estimated prevalence of at least 9.1% by 2025. [24]
More than 30% of the cases were previously undiagnosed, pointing to underestimation of the problem. With ~48 million people affected, diabetes has become one of the main causes of morbidity and mortality in Europe. According to the World Health Organization, ~50% of these patients die of CVDs cardiovascular diseases. It has been well established that surgery in patients with diabetes is associated with longer hospital stay, higher healthcare resource utilization, and greater perioperative mortality. More recently, the emphasis has shifted from diabetes to hyperglycaemia on its own. New-onset hyperglycaemia, as compared with hyperglycaemia in known diabetics, may hold a much higher risk of adverse outcome[25].
Evidence for strict blood glucose control for patients without known diabetes undergoing non-cardiac surgery is largely derived from studies in critically ill patients.[26] the Leuven

prospective randomized controlled study demonstrated major clinical benefits for surgical ICU patients whose blood glucose levels were maintained normal (5.0–5.6mmol/L; 90–100 mg/dL) with intensive insulin therapy, compared with patients who received conventional glucose management and developed hyperglycaemia (8.3–8.9 mmol/L; 150– 160 mg/dL)[27]. These benefits included lower ICU and in-hospital mortality and prevention of several critical illness-associated complications (critical illness polyneuropathy, severe infections, acute renal failure, and prolonged dependency on mechanical ventilation and intensive care). Also, long-term outcome improved, as shown for the cardiac surgery subgroup. Five years later the Leuven group reported findings from the medical ICU, showing prevention of morbidity, but no mortality benefit from intensive glucose control, except in a subgroup requiring critical care for 3 days [28].
Several risk factors for cardiac events after non-cardiac surgery are attenuated with strict blood glucose control in the ICU, including endothelial injury/dysfunction, CRP, and asymmetric dimethylarginine, apart from effects on mitochondrial damage, serum lipid profile, and the cortisol response. No effects, or only marginal ones, were seen on cytokines, coagulation, and fibrinolysis.

Recommendations	**Class[a]**	**Level[b]**
Postoperative prevention of hyperglycaemia (targeting levels at least below 10 mmol/L with intensive insulin therapy is recommended in adults after high risk or complicated major surgery requiring admission to ICU	I	B
Intraoperative prevention of hyperglycaemia with insulin may be considered	II_b	C
Postoperative prevention of hyperglycaemia with insulin after uncomplicated elective surgery may be considered	II_b	C

ICU, Intensive care unit. [a] Class of recommendation. [b] Level of evidence

Table 4. Recommendations on blood glucose control

3. Anaesthetic considerations

The objectives of anaesthesia in patients with aortic stenosis include the prevention of hypotension and any haemodynamic change that will increase the cardiac output.
Normal sinus rhythm must be maintained because the left ventricle is dependant on a properly timed atrial contraction to produce an optimal left ventricular end-diastolic volume. Loss of atrial contraction loosing the atrial kick, as during junctional rhythm or atrial fibrillation may produce a dramatic decrease in stroke volume and blood pressure. The heart rate is important because it determines the time available for ventricular filling, for ejection of the stroke volume, and for coronary perfusion. A sustained increase in heart rate decreases the time for left ventricular filling and ejection and reduces cardiac output. Hypotension reduces coronary blood flow and results in myocardial ischemia and further deterioration in left ventricular function and cardiac output. Aggressive treatment of hypotension is mandatory to prevent cardiogenic shock and/or cardiac arrest. Cardiopulmonary resuscitation is unlikely to be effective in patients with aortic stenosis because it is difficult, if not impossible, to create an adequate stroke volume across a stenotic aortic valve with cardiac compression[1].

3.1 General anaesthesia

General anaesthesia is often selected in preference to epidural or spinal anaesthesia because the sympathetic blockade produced by regional anaesthesia can lead to significant hypotension. [1]Nevertheless controversies do exist as for the careful titration of regional anaesthetic technique that might provide a favourable heamodynamic profile (see below).
Induction of anaesthesia can be with an intravenous induction drug that does not decrease the systemic vascular resistance. An opioid may be useful if left ventricular function is compromised.
Maintenance of anaesthesia with a combination of nitrous oxide and volatile anaesthetic and opioid or by opioid alone. Advisable to avoid drugs depressing the sinus node to preserve atrial contraction which has an important role in the ventricular filling. Drugs that depress sinus node automaticity can produce junctional rhythm and loss of the properly timed atrial contraction. If left ventricular function is impaired, it is prudent to avoid any drugs that can cause additional depression of myocardial contractility. A decrease in systemic vascular resistance is very devastating. Maintenance of anaesthesia with nitrous oxide plus opioid or with opioids alone in high doses is recommended for patients with marked left ventricular dysfunction. Neuromuscular blocking drugs with minimal haemodynamic effects are best used. Intravascular volume should be maintained at normal levels. The onset of junctional rhythm or bradycardia during anaesthesia and surgery requires treatment with glycopyrolate, atropine, or ephedrine. Persistant tachycardia can be treated with ß blockers such as esmolol. Supraventricular tachycardia should be promptly terminated with electrical cardioversion. Lidocaine and defibrillator should be kept available as these patients have a propensity to develop ventricular dysrhythmias[1].

3.2 Epidural block

There is a lack of evidence based guidelines as for the best choice of regional technique to be used in patients with aortic stenosis to provide anaesthesia and analgesia. Patients with hip fractures for instance and cardiac co-morbidities benefit more from epidural analgesia than from opioid analgesia technique in terms of pain and reduced postoperative cardiac events [29]. In major knee surgery it has been demonstrated that earlier rehabilitation can be achieved by using epidural blockade in contrast to i.v. patient controlled morphine [30].
So what is the rule?, When anaesthetizing a patient with aortic stenosis, the haemodynamic goals include avoiding sudden and profound decreases in systemic vascular resistance, maintaining contractility and sinus rhythm and avoiding hypovolaemia and tachycardia (as mentioned earlier in the general anaesthesia section). Epidural blockade facilitate a gradual onset of anaesthesia and sympathetic block, and therefore a sudden and profound decrease in systemic vascular resistance is avoided. With incremental doses of local anaesthetics, an even higher degree of control is attained. Epidural anaesthesia does not affect myocardial contractility and with proper fluid loading, good control of the circulation can be accomplished.
There are some studies e.g. Ho et al. suggested the use of hypotensive epidural anaesthesia in patients with aortic stenosis undergoing total hip replacement and rendered satisfactory results provided that the stenosis is asymptomatic and non-critical. Nevertheless the choice of anaesthesia in such cases should be made on individual basis and in the presence of skilled anaesthetist [31].

3.3 Spinal anaesthesia

Although general anaesthesia is historically considered the anaesthetic of choice for patients with aortic stenosis, Continuous spinal anaesthesia is an attractive alternative for the management of surgery on the lower extremities when used with appropriate invasive monitoring.

Central neuroaxial blockade has been contraindicated in patients with severe aortic stenosis [32-35], because sympathetic blockade produced can rapidly cause a marked decrease in systemic vascular resistance with decreased venous return to the heart and coronary perfusion pressure. Large decreases in systemic vascular resistance, therefore, should be avoided to prevent the catastrophic cycle of hypotension-induced ischemia, subsequent ventricular dysfunction, and worsening hypotension. Indeed, hypotension-induced ischemia with resultant ventricular dysfunction has been described in patients with left ventricular outflow tract obstruction receiving spinal anaesthesia[36]. Recently, several authors have reported greater hemodynamic control achieved with continuous spinal anaesthesia over epidural or single-dose spinal anaesthesia in healthy patients [37, 38].

When regional anaesthesia is selected, epidural rather than spinal anaesthesia is often recommended, but continuous spinal anaesthesia offers many of the advantages of epidural anaesthesia. With the appropriate invasive monitoring, the onset of peripheral sympathetic block develops in a gradual and controlled fashion using continuous spinal anaesthesia. An additional advantage over epidural anaesthesia in that catheter placement is technically easier and aspiration of CSF provides confirmation of correct catheter placement, also the catheter can be left in place like an epidural catheter offering postoperative pain management, minimizing the need for systemic opiates and their attendant risks. However, the potential higher incidence of respiratory depression with spinal versus epidural opiate administration should not be overlooked [39].

Continuous spinal anaesthesia avoids many of the disadvantages of general anaesthesia. In contrast to general anaesthesia, use of a continuous spinal catheter allows patient communication of subjective feelings of distress throughout the operation. In addition, the hemodynamic perturbations of direct laryngoscopy and intubation are avoided with continuous spinal anaesthesia. Moreover, the use of volatile anaesthetics in patients with aortic stenosis may lead to myocardial depression, peripheral vasodilation, and loss of normal atrial systole. Likewise, continuous spinal anaesthesia obviates the need for neuromuscular blockade, which may lead to undesirable fluctuations though newer agents have fewer effects on heart rate.

However, continuous spinal anaesthesia has potential complications:

It should be used with caution in patients in whom a difficult endotracheal intubation is anticipated. Peripheral sympathetic nervous system block produced by continuous spinal anaesthesia may be deleterious in situations of profound blood loss. This is especially true in the setting of aortic stenosis where precipitous decreases in systemic vascular resistance can lead to the catastrophic cycle of hypotension-induced ischemia, subsequent ventricular dysfunction, and worsening hypotension. Aortic stenosis is often complicated by global ventricular hypokinesis and atrial fibrillation. These patients are often anticoagulated and Continuous spinal anaesthesia would be contraindicated. Finally, many of the complications associated with single-dose spinal anaesthesia including postdural puncture headache, persistent paresthesia, low back pain, and risk of infection also apply to continuous spinal anaesthesia.

3.3.1 Pulmonary artery catheter management under continuous spinal anaesthesia

a. Low CVP and PCWP: warrants the administration of e.g. crystalloids or colloids to regain PCWP to the preoperative value, if this measure fails , it is advisable to add a vasoconstrictor to increase the systemic vascular resistance and cardiac filling pressures.
b. In case of crystalloids usage and sudden increase in the PCWP of 3-4 mmHg upon administering 15ml/kg , so the infusion should be stopped immediately.
c. Pulmonary artery catheter carries the advantage of detecting pulmonary hypertension, and left ventricular failure as a result of decreased left ventricular filling and decrease compliance[40]
d. Inotropes should be considered in those with hypotension and high PCWP.

Ephedrine should be used cautiously in the patient with aortic stenosis, as the resultant tachycardia may precipitate myocardial ischemia. With the aide of invasive hemodynamic monitoring, there is a successful induction and maintenance of Continuous spinal anaesthesia in a controlled fashion while maintaining control of the cardiac filling pressures.

3.4 Post-operative pain management

Post-operative pain is a major concern, reported in 5–10% of the patients. It may increase sympathetic drive and delay recovery [41, 42]. The evidence that pain causes organ complications after surgery is less clear. Neuraxial analgesia with local anaesthetics/opioids and/or α2-agonists, i.v. opioids alone or in combination with non-steroidal anti-inflammatory drugs seems to be the most effective. The benefit of invasive analgesic techniques should be weighed against potential dangers. This is of special importance when considering the use of neuraxial blockade in patients under chronic antithrombotic therapy due to increased potential of a neuraxial haematoma. Patient-controlled analgesia is an alternative for postoperative pain relief. Recent meta-analyses of controlled randomized trials show that patient-controlled analgesia has some advantage with regard to patient satisfaction over nurse-controlled or on-demand analgesia[43]. No difference with regard to morbidity or final outcome was demonstrated. Patient-controlled analgesia is an adequate alternative in patients and situations not suited for regional anaesthesia. Routines for follow-up and documentation of effects should be in place[42, 44-46] Non-steroidal anti-inflammatory drugs and the cyclooxygenase- 2 (COX-2) inhibitors have the potential for promoting heart and renal failure as well as thromboembolic events and should be avoided in patients with myocardial ischemia. The COX-2 inhibitors cause less gastrointestinal ulceration and bronchospasm. The final role for these drugs in the treatment of post-operative pain in cardiac patients undergoing non-cardiac surgery has not been defined. The drugs should be avoided in patients with renal and heart failure, elderly patients, patients on diuretics, as well as patients with unstable haemodynamics [47].

4. Obstetric considerations

Management of pregnancy complicated by aortic stenosis requires an accurate assessment of the severity of the disease. Unlike mitral stenosis, clinical symptoms appear very late in the course of the disease. Once patients complain of angina, shortness of breath, or syncope, their risk of sudden death may be out of proportion to the severity of their clinical

symptoms. In the past accurate assessment of the severity of stenosis required cardiac catheterization and significant radiation exposure [48, 49].
Intracardiac pressure gradients cab be accurately measured noninvasively by Doppler echocardiography [50, 51], pressure gradients are calculated by $\Delta P= 4V^2$, where ΔP is the change in pressure and V is the velocity of blood flow determined by Doppler evaluation. Use of the technique has been described in pregnancy, . because pressure gradients are flow-dependant, gradients alone may provide misleading information about the severity of valve narrowing during pregnancy, when cardiac output is increased. In this setting, calculation of aortic valve area provides an index of the stenosis that is independent of changes in transaortic volume flow. Valve area can be determined noninvasively using the Doppler continuity equation [52].
Five principal changes in the cardiovascular system during pregnancy that present unique problems to the parturient with underlying heart disease have been well delineated:

1. 50% increase in intravascular volume that generally peaks by the early to- middle third trimester.
2. Progressive decrease in systemic vascular resistance (SVR) throughout pregnancy, thanks to this mean arterial blood pressure is preserved at normal values, despite a 30%- 40% increase in cardiac output.
3. Marked fluctuations in cardiac output during labour. Pain and apprehension may precipitate an increase in cardiac output to as much as 40%-50% over those levels seen in the late second stage of labour.
4. Each uterine contraction serves as an auto transfusion to the central blood volume, an increase in cardiac output of 10%-25% is seen
5. Hypercoagulability associated with pregnancy and the possible need for appropriate anticoagulation, especially in those patients at increased risk for arterial thrombosis and embolization (prosthetic heart valve).

4.1 General anaesthesia versus other modalities

Improvement of medical and surgical care lead to the decrease in the incidence of rheumatic heart disease and the relative increase in the congenital heat disease in women in the child bearing period. Congenital aortic stenosis is a congenital bicuspid valve leading to valve thickening, subvalvular or tunnel stenosis. In aortic stenosis the coronary blood vessels are distal to the obstruction and are supplied with blood mainly during diastole; in the pregnant state it becomes more difficult to maintain adequate blood flow to the left ventricle because of increasing systolic and end diastolic ventricular pressures. The work of the ventricle is increased and thus it requires a greater coronary artery blood flow; as this cannot be achieved the patient may experience angina and suffer subendocardial ischemia. Regional anaesthesia has been associated with ECG changes of ischemia of multifactorial origin in healthy parturients [53]. The detection of transient ischemia requires capture of ECG data from leads II and V5 and an analysis of changes from control. In spite of the spinal microcatheter technique, colloid infusion and vasopressors intravenously, the patient's systolic blood pressure might decrease. However, it is the diastolic blood pressure which determines myocardial blood flow. The patient with aortic stenosis has a fixed stroke volume and to maintain cardiac output must elevate her heart rate, but this compromises left ventricular filling. The pregnant woman with aortic stenosis is extremely intolerant of change in left ventricular preload. A decrease in preload caused by haemorrhage or associated with regional anaesthesia can produce cardiogenic shock. An increase in preload can precipitate pulmonary oedema. These are acute changes, but they may complicate a more chronic left ventricular hypertrophy which ultimately progresses to congestive cardiac failure. Control over left ventricular preload is less precise with regional techniques because ventilation cannot be manipulated as would be possible with IPPV and filling pressures are less predictable because they depend on fluid load and altered sympathetic nervous system responses. A segmental nerve block from the lowest sacral segment to T4 is necessary by any route to ensure adequate pain relief during Caesarean section and this invariably produces extensive sympathetic block [54]. Moreover, the risk of hypotension cannot be eliminated. Obstetric anaesthetists are agreed that in severe aortic stenosis tachycardia must be prevented, adverse therapeutic events must also be anticipated. If ephedrine is chosen as the vasoconstrictor, it has α and ß effects with a resultant tachycardia which is undesirable in a patient with aortic stenosis. Phenylephrine might be a better choice although it is a pure α agonist [55]. A multidisciplinary approach may be very beneficial in mothers with severe aortic stenosis. The cardiac surgery team in such cases is present during the caesarean section and may take over in case of an emergency [56].

Regardless of the anaesthetic used, blood loss reduces blood volume and to counteract this the uterus contracts and releases additional blood into the circulation. This process is augmented by the use of oxytocin after delivery to ensure uterine contraction and prevent postpartum haemorrhage. One of the deaths reported in the maternal mortality reports describes postpartum cardiac failure exacerbated by oxytocin in a woman with aortic stenosis who required manual removal of the placenta [57]. There is a time and preferably an elective decision, when conversion to general anaesthesia has to be made because of clinical deterioration.

Each patient must be serially assessed during pregnancy by cardiological investigations, including non-invasive Doppler echocardiography and in some cases cardiac catheterisation. The case for general anaesthesia is made on the basis that the avoidance of sympathetic blockade which occurs with regional anaesthesia decreases the risk of significant hypotension following a reduction in systemic vascular resistance. In pregnancy hypotension will compromise not only the maternal myocardium but also the placental blood flow to the foetus. One disadvantage of general anaesthesia is the sympathetic nervous system response to intubation, which can generate tachycardia and hypertension, leading to sudden fluctuations in cardiac output. This can be controlled by induction with a cardio-stable drug followed by a short acting opioid (e.g. alfentanil). Volatile anaesthetic agents also have a direct myocardial depressant effect but this is dose related. In obstetrics, their concentration is limited because of their relaxant effect on the myometrium.

Postoperatively monitoring should continue and it is advised that women with significant cardiac disease should be nursed in a high-dependency unit on the labour ward and cardiac monitoring continued into the puerperium because maternal deaths occur, not uncommonly, 3–5 days postpartum [17]. Postoperative analgesia does not govern the choice of technique for anaesthesia. Patient-controlled analgesia provides satisfactory analgesia after general anaesthesia [58] and by whichever route opioids are administered, respiratory monitoring is required.

4.2 Regional anaesthesia debates

Congenital aortic stenosis has been considered a relative contraindication to pregnancy because of the high maternal mortality (17%) previously reported [59], although this figure has been disputed [60]. The underlying pathophysiology is well known The need to maintain afterload has been extrapolated to suggest that regional analgesia and anaesthesia are contraindicated in pathological states producing a fixed cardiac output.

Authoritative sources state 'high subarachnoid or extradural blockade is contraindicated in patients with cardiovascular disease nevertheless It is possible to provide safe regional anaesthesia for Caesarean section in women with aortic stenosis, but certain conditions must be met.

Firstly, it is essential to identify these women as early as possible in the antenatal period. There is no place for assessing the woman with aortic stenosis a few minutes before she is due to be delivered. Secondly, it is important to make clear written and dated management plans for anaesthesia and delivery in the patient's records. These plans should include provision for emergency delivery and should be amended as necessary during the course of the pregnancy. Regular revision of management plans is important, since deterioration in cardiac status during pregnancy increases maternal risk.

Use of the wedged supine position, or of lateral tilt to ensure displacement of the uterus off the aorta and inferior vena cava, is mandatory during anaesthesia for Caesarean section. It is important to remember that the tilted or wedged position is a compromise between the full lateral position which prevents aortocaval compression and the supine position that the obstetricians would prefer to facilitate surgery. Maintaining the full lateral position until the obstetrician is ready to perform skin incision reduces the risk of haemodynamic instability due to aortocaval compression.

Ultimately there is, of course, no randomised controlled data comparing carefully managed regional anaesthesia with 'cardiac' general anaesthesia for Caesarean section in women with aortic stenosis. All the arguments for and against both techniques are based on anecdotal case reports and assessment of theoretical risks. Multidisciplinary antenatal care of these women is important and should involve senior obstetricians, anaesthetists and cardiologists and regular assessment of cardiac function. Anaesthetic plans for delivery should include provision for the use of invasive monitoring in the peri- and postoperative period and for high-dependency care postoperatively. Both general and regional anaesthesia have significant risks, but incremental induction of either epidural or spinal anaesthesia should be considered a reasonable alternative to general anaesthesia for Caesarean section in the women with aortic stenosis.

5. References

[1] Roberta L Hines,Katherine E Marschall, *Stoelting's Anesthesia and Co-Existing Disease* 5th ed. 2008, Philadelphia: Churchill livingstone.

[2] Rick A. Nishimura.*Aortic Valve Disease.* Circulation, 2002. 106: p. 770-772.

[3] Kennedy KD, Nishimura RA,Holmes DR et al.*Natural history of moderate aortic stenosis.* J Am Coll Cardiol, 1991. 17: 313.

[4] Braunwald E (Ed), *A Textbook of Cardiovascular Medicine (5th Ed) "Valvular heart disease" in Heart Disease*1997, Philadelphia WB Saunders Co. 1007-1076.

[5] Ross J JR,Braunwald E.*Aortic Stenosis.* Circulation, 1968. 38 (suppl V): 61.

[6] ACC/AHA Task Force.*Guidelines for perioperative cardiovascular evaluation for non-cardiac surgery.* Circulation 1996. 93: 1278-1317.

[7] Braunwald E. (ed.).*Heart Disease, 5th edn. Philadelphia: W.B. Saunders.* 1997: 1035-1045.

[8] Connolly HM et al.*Aortic valve replacement for aortic stenosis with severe left ventricular dysfunction. Prognostic indicators.* Circulation, 1997. 95: 2395-2400.

[9] Torsher LC et al.*Risk of patients with severe aortic stenosis undergoing non-cardiac surgery.* Am J Cardiol, 1998. 81: 448-452.

[10] Tang YS. et al.*Aortic stenosis in patients undergoing non-cardiac surgery: the university of Florida experience.* Anesth Analg, 1998. 86: SCA1-SCA124.

[11] Taubert KA Wilson W, Gewitz M, et al.*Prevention of infective endocarditis: guidelines from the American Heart Association: a guideline from the American Heart Association Rheumatic Fever, Endocarditis, and Kawasaki Disease Committee, Council on Cardiovascular Disease in the Young, and the Council on Clinical Cardiology, Council on Cardiovascular Surgery and Anesthesia, and the Quality of Care and Outcomes Research Interdisciplinary Working Group.* Circulation, 2007. 116: 1736 -54.

[12] Biagini A, L'Abbate A, Testa R, *et al.Unreliability of conventional visual electrocardiographic monitoring for detection of transient ST segment changes in a coronary care unit.* Eur Heart J, 1984. 5: 784–791.

[13] Leung JM, O'Kelly B, Browner WS, *et al.Prognostic importance of postbypass regional wall-motion abnormalities in patients undergoing coronary artery bypass graft surgery.* SPI Research Group. Anesthesiology 1989. 71: 16–25.

[14] Leung JM, Voskanian A, Bellows WH, *et al.Automated electrocardiograph ST segment trending monitors: accuracy in detecting myocardial ischemia.* Anesth Analg, 1998. 87: 4–10.

[15] Kaplan JA,King SB 3rd.*The precordial electrocardiographic lead (V5) in patients who have coronary-artery disease.* Anesthesiology, 1976. 45: 570–574.

[16] London MJ, Hollenberg M, Wong MG, *et al.Intraoperative myocardial ischemia: localization by continuous 12-lead electrocardiography.* Anesthesiology, 1988. 69: 232–241.

[17] Landesberg G, Mosseri M, Wolf Y, *et al.Perioperative myocardial ischemia and infarction: identification by continuous 12-lead electrocardiogram with online ST-segment monitoring.* Anesthesiology, 2002. 96: 264–270.

[18] Kertai MD, Boersma E, Klein J, *et al.Longterm prognostic value of asymptomatic cardiac troponin T elevations in patients after major vascular surgery.* Eur J Vasc Endovasc Surg, 2004. 28: 59–66.

[19] Landesberg G, Shatz V, Akopnik I, *et al.Association of cardiac troponin, CK-MB, and postoperative myocardial ischemia with long-term survival after major vascular surgery.* J Am Coll Cardiol 2003. 42: 1547–1554.

[20] Martinez EA, Kim LJ, Faraday N, *et al.Sensitivity of routine intensive care unit surveillance for detecting myocardial ischemia.* Crit Care Med, 2003. 31: 2302–2308.

[21] *Practice guidelines for perioperative transesophageal echocardiography. A report by the American Society of Anesthesiologists and the Society of Cardiovascular Anesthesiologists Task Force on Transesophageal Echocardiography.* Anesthesiology, 1996. 84: 986–1006.

[22] de Vaal JB, de Wilde RBP, van den Berg PCM, *et al.Less invasive determination of cardiac output from the arterial pressure by aortic diameter-calibrated pulse contour.* Br J Anaesth, 2005. 95: 326–331.

[23] Thomas R, H.S. Chadwick Easterling, Catherine M. Otto, *et al. Aortic stenosis in pregnancy.* Obstetrics & gynecology. 72(1): 113-118.

[24] *International Diabetes Federation.* Diabetes atlas, 2006.
[25] Umpierrez GE, Isaacs SD, Bazargan N, *et al. Hyperglycemia: an independent marker of in-hospital mortality in patients with undiagnosed diabetes.* J Clin Endocrinol Metab, 2002. 87: 978–982.
[26] Vanhorebeek I, Langouche L,Van den Berghe G. *Tight blood glucose control with insulin in the ICU: facts and controversies.* Chest 2007. 132: 268–278.
[27] van den Berghe G, Wouters P, Weekers F, *et al. Intensive insulin therapy in the critically ill patients.* N Engl J Med, 2001. 345: 1359–1367.
[28] Van den Berghe G, Wilmer A, Hermans G, *et al. Intensive insulin therapy in the medical ICU.* N Engl J Med, 2006. 354: 449–461.
[29] Matot I, Oppenheim-Edden A,Ratrot R et al. *Preoperative cardiac events in elderly patients with hip fracture randomised to epidural or conventional analgesia.* Anesthesiology, 2003. 98: 156–163.
[30] Capdevila X, Barthelet Y, Biboulet P et al. *Effect of perioperative analgesic technique on the surgical outcome and duration of rehabilitation after major knee surgery.* Anesthesiology, 1999. 91: 8–15.
[31] Ho, Michael C, Beathe, *et al. Hypotensive Epidural Anesthesia in Patients With Aortic Stenosis Undergoing Total Hip Replacement.* Regional Anesthesia & Pain Medicine, 2008. 33 (2): 129–133.
[32] Stoelting RK, Dierdorf SF, *Anesthesia and co-existing disease.* 3rd ed. ed. 1993, New York: Churchill Livingstone.
[33] Stoelting RK, Miller RD, *Basics of anesthesia.* 3rd ed ed. 1994, New York: Churchill Livingstone.
[34] Morgan GE, Mikhail MS, *Clinical anesthesiology.* 1992, Norwalk: Appleton & Lange.
[35] Colough G. *Epidural anesthesia for cesarean delivery in a puarturient with aortic stenosis.* Reg Anesth, 1990. 15: 273-274.
[36] Loubser P, Suh K,Cohen S. *Adverse effects of spinal anesthesia in a patient with idiopathic hypertrophic subaortic stenosis.* Anesth Analg, 1984. 60: 228-30.
[37] Schnider TW, Mueller-Duvsing S, Gerber H, Johr M. *Incremental dosing versus single-dose-spinal anesthesia and hemodynamic stabilitv.* Anesth Analg, 1993. 77: 1174-1178.
[38] Klimscha W, Weinstabl C, Bias W et al. *Continuous spinal anesthesia with a microcatheter and low-dose bupivacaine decreases the hemodynamic effects of centroneuraxis blocks in elderly patients.* Anesth Analg, 1993. 77: 275-280.
[39] Lubenow TR, Ivankovich AD,McCarthy RJ, *Management of acute postoperative pain.* 2nd ed ed. Clinical anesthesia, ed. Barash PG, Cullen BF,Stoelting RK. 1992, Philadelphia: JB Lippincott,.
[40] Skein TM, Thvs DM. *Monitoring the cardiac surgical uatient.* the practice of cardiac anesthesia, ed. Hensley EA Jr,Martin DE. 1990, Boston: Little, Brown and Co.
[41] White PF, Kehlet H. *Postoperative pain management and patient outcome: time to return to work!* Anesth Analg, 2007. 104: 487–489.
[42] Liu SS, Wu CL. *The effect of analgesic technique on postoperative patient-reported outcomes including analgesia: a systematic review.* Anesth Analg, 2007. 105: 789–808.
[43] Polomano RC, Rathmell JP, Krenzischek DA, *et al. Emerging trends and new approaches to acute pain management.* J Perianesth Nurs, 2008. 23 (1 Suppl): S43–S53.
[44] Dolin SJ, Cashman JN,Bland JM.*Effectiveness of acute postoperative pain management: I. Evidence from published data.* Br J Anaesth, 2002. 89: 409–423.

[45] Jorgensen H, Wetterslev J, Moiniche S, *et al. Epidural local anaesthetics versus opioid-based analgesic regimens on postoperative gastrointestinal paralysis, PONV and pain after abdominal surgery.*, in *Cochrane Database Syst Rev.* 2000.

[46] Block BM, Liu SS, Rowlingson AJ, *et al. Efficacy of postoperative epidural analgesia: a meta-analysis.* JAMA, 2003. 290: 2455–2463.

[47] Schug SA, Manopas A. *Update on the role of non-opioids for postoperative pain treatment.* Best Pract Res Clin Anaesthesiol, 2007. 21: 15–30.

[48] Rapaport E. *Natural history of aortic and mitral valve disease.* Am J Cadiol, 1975. 35: 221.

[49] Hossack KF, Heutze JM, Lowe JB et al. *Congenital valvular aortic stenosis-a natural history and assessment of operation.* Br Heart J, 1980. 45: 561.

[50] Hatle L, Angelsen BA, Tromsdal A. *Non invasive asseement of aortic stenosis by Doppler ultrasound.* Br Heart J, 1980. 43: 284.

[51] Currie PJ, Seward JB, Reeder GS et al. *Contiuous-wave Doppler echocardiographic assessemtn of severity of calcific aortic stenosis: A simultaneous Doppler-catheter correlative study in 100 adult patients.* Circulation, 1985. 71: 1162.

[52] Otto CM, Pearlman AS, Comess KA et al. D*etermination of the stenotic aortic valve area in adults using Doppler echocardiography.* J Am Coll Cadiol 1986. 7: 509.

[53] Burton A, Camman W. *Electrocardiographic changes during cesarean section: a review.* Internal Journal of Obstetric Anesthesia, 1996. 5: 47–53.

[54] Hall PA, Bennet A, Wilkes MP, *et al. Spinal anaesthesia for Caesarean section: comparison of infusions of phenylephrine and ephedrine.* British Journal of Anaesthesia, 1994. 73: 471–474.

[55] Moran D, Perillo M, LaParta R, *et al. Phenylephrine in the prevention of hypotension following spinal anesthesia for Cesarean delivery.* Journal of Clinical Anesthesia 1991. 3: 301–305.

[56] Ghosh S, Marton S. *Anaesthetic management for cesarean delivery in a patient with severe aortic stenosis and severe obesity.* Obes Surg, 2011. 21: 264-6.

[57] *Report on Confidential Enquiry into Maternal Deaths in England and Wales 1979–1981* HMSO 1980.

[58] Howell PR, Gambling DR, Pavy T, *et al. Patient controlled analgesia following Caesarean section under general anaesthesia: a comparison of fentanyl with morphine.* Canadian Journal of Anaesthesia, 1995. 42: 41–45.

[59] Arias F, Pineda J. *Aortic stenosis and pregnancy.* Journal of Reproductive Medicine 1978. 20: 229–232.

[60] Shime J, Mocarski EJM, Hastings D, *et al. Congenital heart disease in pregnancy: short- and long-term implications.* American Journal of Obstetrics and Gynecology, 1987. 156: 313–322.

4

Operative Management – Patient-Prosthesis Mismatch

Koji Tsutsumi
Division of Cardiovascular Surgery, National Hospital Organization Tokyo Medical Center, Tokyo, Japan

1. Introduction

The main objective of aortic valve replacement (AVR) is to relieve left ventricular (LV) burden and normalized LV mass (LVM). During AVR, many surgeons make final decision to select the size of the prosthetic valve based on intraoperative measurement. It is ideal to place an aortic prosthesis that is appropriately sized to the patient. However, this is not always possible owing to insufficient aortic annular dimensions. Patients receive a prosthesis that is too small in relation to their body size have persistent abnormally high gradients across the valve and may even show deterioration of symptoms and hemodynamics after AVR. Rahimtoola first described the concept of patient-prosthesis mismatch (PPM), which was defined as existing "when the effective prosthetic valve area, after insertion into the patient, is less than that of a normal valve" [1]. The optimal prosthetic valve should have several characteristics, including a sufficiently large effective orifice area (EOA) with a reduced transvalvular pressure gradient around zero, long-term durability, and anticoagulability. There is no optimal, commercially available prosthesis. The normal aortic valve has 3.0-4.5 cm^2 of EOA, but this is rarely achieved with present commercially available prostheses, which means that the result of AVR may be suboptimal in many patients. In general, PPM is considered to be present when an indexed EOA (IEOA) adjusted for body surface area (BSA) is <0.85 cm^2/m^2 [2-4]. Although, many studies have shown that PPM adversely affects survival and postoperative cardiac function [2-4], many studies contradict these findings [5-12]. Thus, there is considerable controversy regarding the effects of PPM on survival and postoperative recovery of cardiac functions. Patients with a small aortic annulus is still challenging and usually require several surgical measures to minimize the PPM, such as use of supra-annular implantation technique, high-performance prostheses, aortic annular enlargement, or the Ross procedure. The surgical strategy is determined based on the individual patient's conditions, including the size of the aortic annulus, patient's age, BSA, preoperative activity level, and ventricular function. Avoiding the risk of severe PPM defined as an IEOA <0.70 cm^2/m^2, which may prevent symptom resolution and regression of left ventricular hypertrophy and may adversely affect late cardiac events and survival, must always be considered by taking appropriate surgical strategies, but, it is more important to consider whether the benefits of avoiding PPM overcome the drawbacks of other complicated measures in each individual patient.

2. General consideration

2.1 Left ventricular-aortic pressure gradients

Gradients are minimal after AVR with aortic and pulmonary autograft or allograft but are present after mechanical or bioprosthetic AVR in virtually all patients. Their magnitude varies greatly, determined primarily by the characteristics of the prosthesis itself, the size of the prosthesis relative to the size of the patient, and the cardiac output (whether the study was done during rest or exercise). Smaller-sized stented bioprostheses and mechanical prostheses can result with residual transvalvular gradients. In clinical, conventional mechanical prostheses and bioprostheses larger than the 21-mm size can provide satisfactory performance in most adults. On the other hand, the small resting gradients associated with conventional 19-mm prostheses may become 30 to 50 mmHg during periods of increased cardiac output. However, in patients with small body size, when the patient's body surface area is less than 1.5 m^2, (with their smaller cardiac output) conventional 19-mm devices may perform satisfactorily. The relationship between peak left ventricular-aortic gradient and prosthesis size was mainly dependent on the patient's BSA.

3. Definitions of PPM

In general, PPM is considered to be present when an IEOA is $<0.85\ cm^2/m^2$ [2-4]. IEOA has been reported as an index that correlates with the severity of PPM [2-6]. In present chapter, mild to moderate PPM is defined as when an IEOA of $\geq 0.70 cm^2/m^2$ and $<0.85\ cm^2/m^2$, and severe PPM is defined as when an IEOA of less than $0.69\ cm^2/m^2$.

3.1 Effect of PPM on valve related event and survival

Blais et al. reported the results of 2981 patients who underwent AVR with a stented bioprosthesis [3]. According to the literature, patients with an EOAI $<0.75\ cm^2/m^2$ was a significant risk factor for increased operative mortality and valve related deaths during the follow-up period. Medalion et al. reported the long-term results of 892 patients who underwent AVR [7]. Moderate PPM had no influence on survival, but advanced age, chronic obstructive pulmonary disease, chronic renal failure, and smoking were significant risk factors. Urso et al. showed improvement in postoperative NHYA class and regression of LVMI during long-term follow-up in patients who underwent AVR with a 19-mm mechanical valve [12]. We also showed that PPM with an EOAI $\geq 0.75\ cm^2/m^2$ but $<0.85\ cm^2/m^2$ has no effect on operative, short-term, and long-term survival and the effect of PPM with an IEOA $<0.75\ cm^2/m^2$ on survival appeared to decrease over time [11]. Surviving patients with an IEOA $<0.75\ cm^2/m^2$ showed good long-term survival. Although, the effect of PPM on postoperative valve related event and late survival could not be definitively determined due to lack of a radomised large population and long-term follow-up study, in some patients with mild to moderate PPM could be tolerable in patients with preserved LV function without any impact on overall survival.

3.2 The significance of IEOA

Recently, aortic valve stenosis has become the leading type of valvular heart disease in developed countries, and such stenosis is no longer caused by rheumatic fever but is due to aging. Consequently, the age of candidates for AVR have increased markedly and have more risk factors and complications. These findings suggest that surgery becomes more complicated. Moreover, most patients with aortic stenosis have calcific aortic valve sclerosis, which typically becomes clinically significant in seventh or eighth decade of life. Therefore, the incidence of patients with a small aortic annulus with calcification is also increasing, especially in Japan. This may result in increasing number of patients with PPM after AVR. Some previous studies have reported that the risk factors for AVR patients with aortic stenosis developing PPM postoperatively are female gender and advanced age [2-4, 10]. Aortic annular enlargement procedures should achieve the optimal measurements to prevent PPM, but these procedures lengthen the cardiopulmonary bypass and cross clamp times, increasing the surgical risks. Several reports demonstrated that aortic annular enlargement is related to increased operative mortality [15]. In such circumstance, surgery should be restricted to the minimum necessary. The EOA of commercially available prosthetic valves was only 49 - 66% that of a normal aortic valve [1-9]. PPM patients have significantly higher persistent pressure gradients across the valve prosthesis than patients without significant PPM. It is well recognized that the transvalvular pressure gradient increases exponentially with a decrease in prosthetic valve EOA [4]. A small decrease in EOA results in a relatively large increase in the transvalvular pressure gradient. Several reports demonstrated that PPM increases LV workload due to the residual pressure gradient, which prevents regression of LVM and increases operative mortality and valve-related events [1-6]. The definition of the threshold degree of severe PPM that must be avoided due to an adverse effect on survival is important. Tasca et al. reported that there was a positive correlation between LVM and IEOA, and patients with an IEOA <0.80 cm^2/m^2 showed inadequate regression of LVM after AVR. Moreover, an inadequate regression of LVM positively affected the rate of valve-related events after AVR and patients with an IEOA <0.70 cm^2/m^2 showed regression of indexed LVM; LVMI (LVM adjusted for BSA), but LVMI increased again during the follow-up period [6]. This phenomenon suggests that AVR contributes to decreasing the pressure gradient across the valve to less than that of the preoperative state. Decreased workload to the left ventricle can lead to regression of LVMI in the postoperative acute phase. However, LV workload remains high after AVR due to persistent PPM, which may increase LVM again during the follow-up period. On the other hand, many studies have been reported that mild to moderate PPM appears to have little or no effect on postoperative recovery of cardiac function, late cardiac events and survival[5-12]. Such degree of PPM may be acceptable in not only elderly patients but also younger patients[7]. We also reported that the postoperative peak pressure gradient across the prosthesis was significantly higher in patients with PPM than in patients without PPM, but postoperative cardiac function, including LV function, LVMI, and NYHA class, improved in all patients despite having PPM; the degree of improvement in cardiac function in patients with PPM compared favorably to that in patients without PPM [11]. Avoiding the risk of severe PPM, must always be considered, but, it is more important to consider whether the benefits of avoiding PPM overcome the drawbacks of other complicated measures in each individual patient. There is controversy about applying a unified standard for avoiding PPM to every patients requiring AVR regardless of their age and preoperative condition. The current perception of PPM based on the value of IEOA may need to be reconsidered for select populations. Based on these findings, IEOA ranges from 0.70 cm^2/m^2 to 0.75 cm^2/m^2 may be a lower tolerable threshold limit [5-11].

3.3 Optimal surgery for patients with advanced age

In general, elderly patients have decreased physiological reserve, and unexpected bleeding could occur during the operation due to tissue fragility, which may result in difficulty achieving hemostasis. In such circumstances, surgery should be restricted to the minimum necessary to obtain improved performance. Elderly patients with a short stature, in a relatively inactive, if the patient's LV function remains preserved, then it is not necessary to replace the valve with a larger prosthesis to ensure an IEOA ≥0.85 cm^2/m^2, or even to perform additional aortic root enlargement. PPM with an IEOA <0.85 cm^2/m^2 and ≥0.70 cm^2/m^2 could be tolerable without any impact on overall survival[5-11].

4. Introduction of high-performance prostheses

4.1 Prosthetic performance

In contrast to other risk factors, PPM can be largely avoided with the use of a prospective strategy at the time of operation. Determine patient's BSA and estimate the minimum required prosthetic size for patient. Confirm the indicated sizer pass through the patient's aortic annulus. Currently, high-performance mechanical or bioprosthetic valves that have a larger EOA than those of corresponding labeled sizes of conventional prostheses have been introduced [13, 14]. These valves have a low incidence of PPM without performing annular enlargement, especially in the small valve sizes. In recent years, patients who require AVR are becoming older and thus have more risk factors and complications. In such circumstances, operative invasiveness should be minimized, and there is a tendency to perform isolated AVR with a high-performance prosthesis instead of performing aortic annular enlargement. However, there are several drawbacks and advantages in high-performance prostheses. Stentless prosthesis can avoid PPM with excellent hemodynamics, but implantation of this prosthesis is more complicated than that of standard AVR. SJM Regent valve has a larger EOA than the corresponding same-labeled size of SJM standard valve. On the other hand, the thickness of the external sewing ring of SJM Regent valve is very thin, so that considerable concern might exist about the fit between the external sewing ring and the native aortic annulus. Making an appropriate choice with regard to the prosthesis is important.

Table 1 shows currently available several types of high-performance mechanical prostheses, which includes the conventional type of St. Jude Medical Standard aortic valve (Medtronic, Minneapolis, MN, USA) for comparison; St. Jude Medical Hemodynamic Plus; St. Jude Medical Regent; and ATS AP 360 (ATS Medical Inc, Minneapolis, MN, USA). For each type and size of prosthetic valve, the estimates of the prostheses' EOAs were obtained from the manufacturers' instructions.

The spectrum of biological valve substitutes for the small aortic annulus includes stented and stentless porcine valves, stented pericardial valves, aortic or pulmonary homografts, and pulmonary autografts. Table 2 shows currently available several types of high-performance bioprostheses, which includes the conventional type of Carpentier-Edwards Perimount aortic valve (Edwards Lifesciences, Irvine, CA, USA) for comparison; Carpentier-Edwards Perimount Magna; Mosaic Porcine Bioprosthesis (Medtronic, Minneapolis, MN, USA); and Freestyle Aortic Root Bioprosthesis (Medtronic). For each type and size of prosthetic valve, the estimates of the prostheses' EOAs were obtained from the manufacturers' instructions.

Prosthesis									
Size (mm)	**16**	**17**	**18**	**19**	**20**	**21**	**22**	**23**	**25**
SJM Standard				1.00		1.30		1.60	1.80
SJM HP		1.00		1.30		1.60			
SJM Regent		1.30		1.70		2.00		2.50	2.60
ATS AP360	1.20		1.50		1.70		2.10		

Results are the effective orifice area (cm^2)

SJM, St. Jude Medical; HP, Hemodynamic Plus;
ATS, ATS Medical

Table 1. Effective orifice area of each high-performance mechanical prosthesis

Prosthesis						
Size (mm)	**19**	**21**	**23**	**25**	**27**	**29**
CEP	1.28	1.69	1.87	1.89		
CEP Magna	1.58	1.90	2.07	2.33		
Mosaic	1.20	1.30	1.50	1.80	2.00	2.10
Freestyle-s	1.10	1.40	1.60	2.00	2.40	2.70
Freestyle-f	1.20	1.40	1.70	2.10	2.40	2.70

Results are the effective orifice area (cm^2)

CEP, Carpentier-Edwards Perimount

Freestyle-s, Freestyle subcoronary

Freestyle-f, Freestyle full root

Table 2. Effective orifice area of each high-performance bioprosthesis

5. Surgery for small aortic annulus

Ideally, a patient with a small aortic annulus should be identified preoperatively, so that alternative measures, such as an aortic root-enlarging procedure or a selection of high-performance prosthesis, might be considered. Occasionally, the precise size of the aortic annulus cannot be determined until the time of operation.

5.1 Supra-annular implantation

One-size up prosthesis implantation can be allowed using supra-annular position or single suture technique. Other approach to the slightly smaller aortic annulus is to implant prosthesis at a slight angle to the plane of the annulus [16]. After the sutures are placed in the annulus for a supra-annular position, they are passed through the sewing ring and lowered into place so that the sewing ring is below the left and right coronary arteries but angled upward at the noncoronary sinus. The left and right annulus sutures are tied first, thereby securing the sewing ring to the annulus below the left and right coronary ostia. The sutures that correspond to the noncoronary annulus are tied last, allowing the valve to ride slightly above the annulus in this region.

5.2 Aortic root enlargement

Annular enlargement procedures are alternatives for those patients in whom a prosthesis being implanted is too small in relation to body size (at least 19-mm cannot be implanted). Although, Manouguian's or the Nicks procedure for annular enlargement may increase operative risks, these procedures can allow larger prosthesis implantation in patients with small aortic annulus [15]. Among surviving patients, aortic annular enlargement improved long-term outcome. Recently, with the introduction of high-performance prostheses and changes in the patient's age group, the need for aortic annular enlargement has decreased dramatically in our clinical practice.

5.3 Nicks procedure

Nicks et al. reported a technique for the enlargement of a small aortic root by an operation whereby the small aortic root has been enlarged by insertion of a Dacron fabric gusset that it will accommodate a larger sized prosthesis [17]. In many cases, enlarging the annulus by 2-4 mm may be sufficient. One technique associated with minimal increase in morbidity is to create a posterior annular split at noncoronary cusps, leaving the anterior mitral leaflet and the left atrium intact. The aortic incision is carried downwards posteriorly through the noncoronary aortic sinus across the aortic annulus as far as the origin of the mitral valve, just above the confluence of the intervalvular trigone, left atrial wall, and mitral annulus. A tongue of Dacron fabric is sutured down to the fibrous origin of the mitral annulus.

5.4 Manoughian procedure

Manoughian et al. reported when greater annular enlargement is desired, a posterior incision is made at the commissure between the left and noncoronary cusp and extended through the annulus and the intervalvular trigone into the center of the anterior mitral leaflet [18]. The free edge and body of the anterior leaflet remain intact. The left atrium, which is entered at its attachment with the aortic root, can be opened further to facilitate exposure.

An elliptical patch is used to close the defect in the anterior mitral leaflet. Interrupted horizontal mattress sutures are placed in the annulus and also through the patch. The prosthesis is thus seated, using the patch as part of the annulus. The incision in the left atrial wall is closed by continuous sutures by incorporating the atrial edges as the patch is sutured to the defect in the anterior mitral leaflet. The superior portion of the patch is incorporated into the aortotomy closure. Mitral regurgitation due to distortion of the anterior mitral leaflet may occur.

5.5 Konno procedure

Patients with congenital aortic stenosis have associated hypoplasia of the aortic annulus. In such cases, valvotomy is of limited value, and standard AVR is unfeasible because of the narrow aortic root. In such cases, Konno procedure is indicated [19]. The procedure consists of a longitudinal incision in the aortic septum placed in the midportion of the two coronary ostia, a vertical incision in the outflow tract of the right ventricle to join the septal incision, AVR with prosthetic valve, and patch reconstruction of the outflow tracts of both ventricles by means of two layers of a fusiform Dacron patch.

5.6 Stentless bioprosthesis

The stentless porcine bioprosthesis has become increasingly popular, because stentless xenograft valves have several advantages over the traditional stent mounted tissue valves. Notably, stented xenograft valves are intrinsically obstructive due to the space occupied by the stent and sewing ring. For a given external diameter, the internal diameter of the stentless valve is 2 to 4 mm larger than a stent mounted xenograft valve due to lack of a stent. This translates to an ability to place a bioprosthesis with a greater EOA, reduce mean transvalvular gradients, and results in greater regression of LV hypertrophy compared to the stented bioprosthesis. An increased understanding of the functional anatomy of the aortic root has reinforced the concept of the dynamic relationships among the valve cusps, annulus, sinus of Valsalva, and sinotubular junction. The use of a stentless valve maintains these interactions resulting in improved hemodynamic performance. Stentless valves can be implanted in the subcoronary position, as an aortic root replacement, or as a root inclusion. Although, subcoronary implantation, aortic root replacement, and root inclusion are similar to techniques, implantation of a stentless xenograft aortic valve is technically more difficult than a stented valve but easier than an allograft used in the subcoronary position. Two valves approved for use by the United States Food and Drug Administration are the Toronto SPV (St. Jude, Minneapolis, MN) and the Freestyle valve (Medtronic, Minneapolis, MN). The Toronto SPV is comprised of the valve and supporting aortic wall only, and is designed as a subcoronary implant.

5.7 Apicoaortic bypass

Surgical relief of LV outflow tract obstruction may be difficult to achieve by conventional methods. Creation of a LV "vent" was accomplished by the anastomosis of a valved conduit graft from LV apex to the abdominal aorta [20]. A median sternotomy incision is made and extended into the linear alba after the decision is made to insert the conduit. The supraceliac aorta is exposed and clamped while the anastomosis is performed. During temporary cardiopulmonary bypass a plug of myocardium is removed from the apex of the left ventricle. The rigid inlet tube attached to a sewing ring and fabric graft is sutured to the ventricular ostium. The graft passed into the abdomen through an incision in the diaphragm and the composite conduit is anastomosed end to end fashion.

5.8 Ross procedure

The Ross Procedure is a type of specialized aortic valve surgery where the patient's diseased aortic valve is replaced with his or her own pulmonary valve [21]. The pulmonary valve is then replaced with cryopreserved pulmonary allograft. In children and young adults, or older particularly active patients, this procedure offers several advantages over traditional aortic valve replacement with manufactured prostheses. Longevity of the pulmonary autograft in the aortic position is superior to bioprostheses such as porcine valves, which tend to degenerate after only a few years in patients under 35 years of age. Furthermore, anticoagulation is not required as with mechanical valves. Thus, individuals can lead an active life without the risks associated with anticoagulation therapy. This is especially important for women of child bearing age needing aortic valve replacement, as anticoagulation is contraindicated in pregnancy. However, lifelong follow-up for pulmonary autograft, implanted allograft, and the ascending aortic diameter must be required.

6. Conclusions

PPM with an IEOA <0.70 cm^2/m^2 should always be avoided. This degree of PPM adversely affects operative mortality and postoperative recovery of cardiac functions. However, in some cases, PPM with an IEOA <0.85 cm^2/m^2 and ≥ 0.70 cm^2/m^2 could be acceptable in patients with preserved LV function without any impact on overall survival. The current perception of PPM may need to be reconsidered with respect to the unified standard regardless of each patient's condition. On the other hand, introduction of high-performance prostheses reduces the incidence of PPM without performing annular enlargement, especially in the small valve sizes. Making an appropriate choice, including the surgical strategy and the prosthesis, based on each individual patient's preoperative condition is very important.

7. References

[1] Rahimtoola SH. The problem of prosthesis-patient mismatch. *Circulation* 1978; 58:20-4.

[2] Pibarot P et al. Impact of prosthesis-patient mismatch on hemodynamic and symptomatic status, morbidity and mortality after aortic valve replacement with a bioprosthetic heart valve. *J Heart Valve Dis* 1998; 7:211-8.

[3] Blais C et al. Impact of valve prosthesis-patient mismatch on short-term mortality after aortic valve replacement. *Circulation* 2003; 108:983-8.

[4] Pibarot P et al. Hemodynamic and clinical impact of prosthesis-patient mismatch in the aortic valve position and its prevention. *J Am Coll Cardiol* 2000; 36:1131-41.

[5] Carrel T et al. Early in vivo experience with the Hemodynamic Plus St. Jude Medical heart valves in patients with narrowed aortic annulus. *Ann Thorac Surg* 1996; 61:1418-22.

[6] Tasca G et al. Impact of the improvement of valve area achieved with aortic valve replacement on the regression of left ventricular hypertrophy in patients with pure aortic stenosis. *Ann Thorac Surg* 2005; 79:1291-6.

[7] Penta de Peppo A et al. Small functional size after mechanical aortic valve replacement: No risk in young to middle-age patients. *Ann Thorac Surg* 2005; 79:1915-20.

[8] Medalion B et al. Aortic valve replacement: Is valve size important? *J Thorac Cardiovasc Surg* 2000; 119:963-74.

[9] Koch CG et al. Impact of prosthesis-patient size on functional recovery after aortic valve replacement. *Circulation* 2005; 111:3221-9.

[10] Fuster RG et al. Patient-prosthesis mismatch in aortic valve replacement: really tolerable? *Eur J Cardio Thorac Surg* 2005; 27:441-9.

[11] Tsutsumi K et al. Effect of prosthesis-patient mismatch on survival after aortic valve replacement using mechanical prostheses in patients with aortic stenosis. *Gen Thorac Cardiovasc Surg* 2008; 56:577-83.

[12] Ruel M et al. Prosthesis-patient mismatch after aortic valve replacement predominantly affects patients with preexisting left ventricular dysfunction: Effect on survival, freedom from heart failure, and left ventricular mass regression. *J Thorac Cardiovasc Surg* 2006; 131:1036-41.

[13] Urso S et al. Is patient-prosthesis mismatch an independent risk factor for early and mid-term overall mortality in adult patients undergoing aortic replacement? *Interac CardioVasc Thorac Surg* 2009; 9:510-8.

[14] Vitale N et al. Clinical evaluation of St. Jude Medical Hemodynamic Plus versus standard aortic valve prostheses; the Italian multicenter, prospective, randomized study. *J Thorac Cardiovasc Surg* 2001; 122:691-8.

[15] Bach DS et al; SJM Regent Study Group. Hemodynamics and early performance of the St. Jude Medical Regent aortic valve prosthesis. *J Heart Valve Dis* 2001; 10:436-42.

[16] Sommers KE et al. Aortic valve replacement with patch enlargement of the aortic annulus. *Ann Thorac Surg* 1997; 63:1608-12.

[17] Olin CL et al. Optimal insertion technique for the Bjork-Shiley valve in the narrow aortic ostium. *Ann Thorac Surg 1983;36:567-82.*

[18] Nicks R et al. hypoplasia of the aortic root. *Thorax* 1970;25:339-46.

[19] Manouguian S et al. Patch enlargement of the aortic valve ring by extending the aortic incision into the anterior mitral leaflet. *J Thorac Cardiovasc Surg* 1979;78:402-12.

[20] Konno S et al. A new method for prosthetic valve replacement in congenital aortic stenosis associated with hypoplasia of the aortic valve ring. *J Thorac Cardiovasc Surg* 1975;70:909-17.

[21] Cooley DA et al. Surgical treatment of left ventricular outflow tract obstruction with apicoaortic valved conduit. *Surgery*1976;80:674-80.

[22] Ross DN. Replacement of the aortic and mitral valves with a pulmonary autograft. *Lancet* 1967;2:956-8.

5

Patient-Prosthesis Mismatch After Aortic Valve Replacement

Wauthy Pierre and Malekzadeh-Milani Sophie G.
Brugmann University Hospital,Brussels, Belgium

1. Introduction

Aortic valve replacement (AVR) is the treatment of choice for the majority of symptomatic adults with aortic valve stenosis. Despite improvements in bioprosthesis durability and reduction of complication rate (both thrombotic and hemorrhagic) of mechanical prosthesis, the ideal valve prosthesis is still elusive.
The hemodynamic performance of the native cardiac valve still outrivals that of prosthesis. In a way, any implanted cardiac prosthesis valve is stenotic compared to its native counterpart.
The concept of patient-prosthesis mismatch (PPM) was first described by Rahimtoola in 1978. According to this author, PPM exists whenever the effective orifice area (EOA) of an implanted prosthesis is inferior to the normal human valve (Rahimtoola, 1978). It can thus be said that, in this situation, the implanted prosthesis is stenotic compared to the normal native valve. On echocardiographic evaluation, those patients show a high transprothetic gradient despite a normal prosthetic valve function. The smaller the prosthetic valve EOA and the larger the patients body surface area, the more severe will be the mismatch and the observed gradient. Thus, the most useful definition and quantification of PPM is the ratio EOA/body surface area (EOA indexed to body surface area).
The prevalence of moderate PPM varies in different studies from 20 to 70% of cases whereas severe PPM is present in 2 to 11% (Pibarot and Dumesnil, 2006). PPM is thus a frequently encountered hemodynamic problem after aortic valve replacement.

2. Definition of the patient-prosthesis mismatch

Theoretically, an observed high transprosthetic gradient can result from two distinct situations. First, a "pathologic" obstruction can result from malfunction of the prosthesis: the motion of a mechanical prosthesis can be hindered by thrombus or pannus while deterioration of a bioprosthesis can result in rigidification of its leaflets. Besides, endocarditis can cause obstructive vegetation masses limiting leaflet motion. Second, a "physiologic" obstruction exists when the normally functioning prosthetic valve has too small EOA to accommodate the cardiac output without generating too much of a gradient. In all cases, a component of perivalvular obstacle must be excluded before blaming the prosthesis.
Patient-prosthesis mismatch is present when the effective orifice area (EOA) of a prosthetic valve is too small in relation to the body size of the patient. The hemodynamic consequence is the higher than expected gradient observed through a normally functioning prosthetic valve.

The clinical significance of PPM is diversely appreciated in the literature. For some authors, the consequences are minimal whereas for others, more severe PPM can even affect postoperative survival. This discordance is due in fact to different ways of evaluating EOA. As a whole, studies based on an in vivo evaluation of the indexed EOA tend to report clinical implications (Blais et al., 2003, Kulik et al., 2006, Ruel et al., 2006, Ruel et al., 2004, Tasca et al., 2006). In the contrary, the in vitro evaluation of the indexed EOA tends to underestimate clinical implications of PPM (Koch et al., 2005).
The transvalvular gradient (TVG) is determined by the hydraulic equation:

$$TVG=Q^2/(kxEOA^2) \tag{1}$$

Q stands for flow and k is a constant.
This equation shows that the transvalvular gradient is directly related to the square of transvalvular flow and inversely related to the square to the valve EOA (Effective Orifice Area of the valve). The flow is dependent on cardiac output which is at rest related to body surface area (BSA).
Mismatch can occur in aortic position and in mitral position. We will focus on the aortic PPM.
There is a large body of evidence that the best variable to evaluate transvalvular gradient at rest and during exercise is the indexed EOA: EOA is divided by the body surface area (Dumesnil and Pibarot, 2011, Pibarot et al., 2000, Zoghbi et al., 2009, Bleiziffer et al., 2007). This indexed EOA is the key factor used to define mismatch. Pibarot showed that the relation between transvalvular gradient and indexed EOA is curvilinear and that the gradient increases exponentially when the indexed EOA is inferior to 0.8 to 0.9 cm^2/m^2 (Pibarot and Dumesnil, 2000). The relation of the transvalvular gradient and indexed EOA are curvilinear at rest (Figure 1) and in stress conditions (Figure 2).

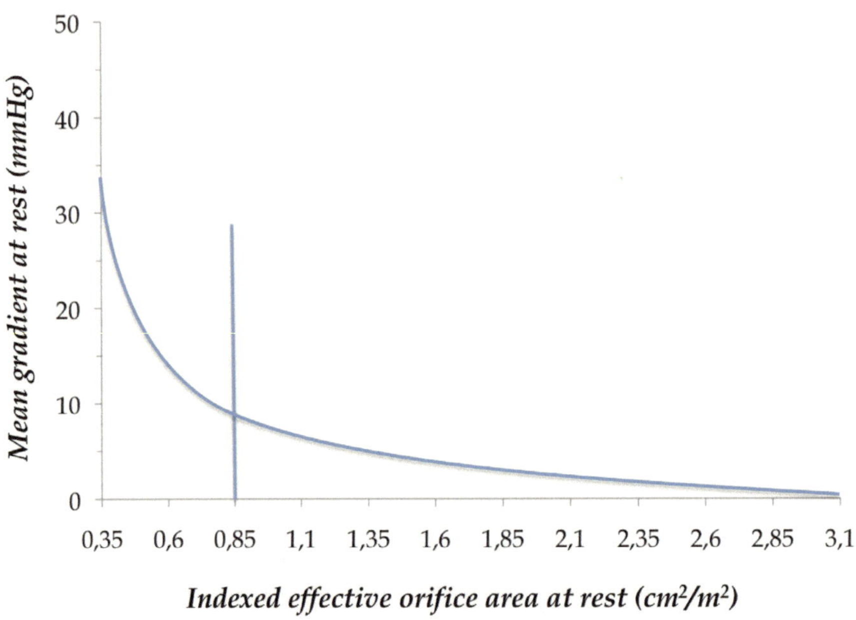

Fig. 1. Curvilinear relation of the gradient and indexed EOA at rest.

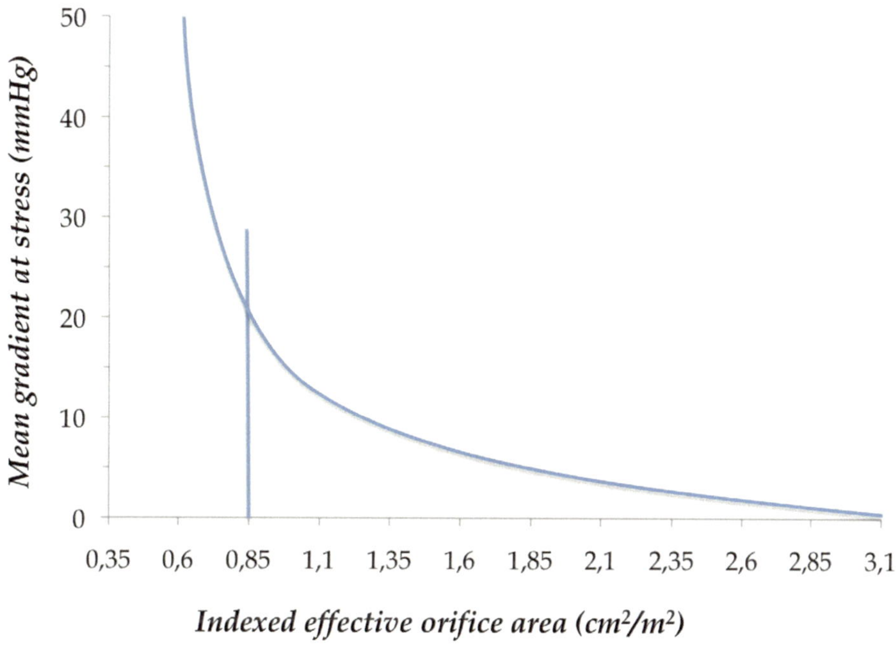

Fig. 2. Curvilinear relation of the gradient and indexed EOA at stress.

Based in this chart, PPM is considered present if indexed EOA (iEOA) is < 0,85 cm^2/m^2. It is graded moderate if the iEOA stands between 0,65 and 0,85 cm^2/m^2 and severe if less than 0,65 cm2/m2 (Pibarot and Dumesnil, 2000, Pibarot and Dumesnil, 2006).

3. Identification of PPM

Patient-prosthesis mismatch has several major clinical impacts described below and these impacts increase proportionally with the severity of PPM (Blais et al., 2003, Milano et al., 2002). It is thus important to quantify the severity of this hemodynamic situation.
PPM can be diagnosed and quantified on echocardiography when iEOA is measured. It can also be predicted or estimated at the time of surgery by using the projected EOA derived from in vivo studies and available for each type and size of prosthetic valve as illustrated in Table 1.
Echocardiography is the gold standard for the non invasive evaluation of prosthetic valve function. It is more demanding to perform and interpret data from a prosthetic valve compared to native valve. However, EOA can be calculated on echocardiography and with some other useful measurements lead to the diagnosis of PPM.
The degree of obstruction, the start point of the valve assessment, varies with the type and the size of the valve. To some extend every prosthetic valve is at least partly restrictive resulting in a mild acceleration though the prosthetic orifice. It may be difficult to differentiate obstructive hemodynamic conditions due to valve design from those of mild obstruction due to prosthetic dysfunction and from PPM.
A full echocardiography study is mandatory. The report should include height, weight, BSA, blood pressure, age, gender and the type of prosthetic valve implanted.

	Medtronic Freestyle®					
Prosthesis size	**19**	**21**	**23**	**25**	**27**	**29**
EOA (cm^2/m^2)	1,15	1,35	1,48	2	2,32	
BSA (m^2)						
1	1,15	1,35	1,48	2,00	2,32	
1,1	1,04	1,23	1,34	1,82	2,11	
1,2	0,96	1,12	1,23	1,67	1,93	
1,3	0,88	1,04	1,14	1,54	1,78	
1,4	0,82	0,96	1,06	1,43	1,66	
1,5	0,77	0,90	0,99	1,33	1,55	
1,6	0,72	0,84	0,92	1,25	1,45	
1,7	0,68	0,79	0,87	1,18	1,36	
1,8	0,64	0,75	0,82	1,11	1,29	
1,9	0,60	0,71	0,78	1,05	1,22	
2	0,57	0,67	0,74	1,00	1,16	
2,1	0,55	0,64	0,70	0,95	1,10	
2,2	0,52	0,61	0,67	0,91	1,05	
2,3	0,50	0,59	0,64	0,87	1,01	
2,4	0,48	0,56	0,62	0,83	0,97	
2,5	0,46	0,54	0,59	0,80	0,93	

Table 1. Indexed EOA by prosthesis sizes. Data from the literature (Blais et al., 2003).

3.1 2D echocardiography

The valve should be carefully imaged in 2D (presence of calcification, thrombus, leaflets motion). This can be difficult due to the artifacts created by the valve itself and due to the sometimes calcified aorta. Cardiac chambers have to be evaluated with a specific attention to the left ventricle (LV). Indeed LV mass, thickness, systolic and diastolic function need to be assessed. The aortic root and ascending aorta have to be measured as well as the left ventricle outflow (LVO) tract. This measure is important because it is used in the EOA measurement. It should be measured in parasternal long axis view or in a modified lower parasternal location to avoid the artifacts of the prosthesis. In EOA evaluation, artifacts induced by the prosthesis structure are the most frequent source of error.

3.2 Doppler echocardiography

The second part of the study is Doppler echocardiography. Several items need to be determined in order to rule out or diagnosed PPM:

1. Peak velocity, gradient and Velocity Time Integral (VTI) of the jet;
2. Effective Orifice Area;
3. Doppler Velocity Index;
4. Evaluation of the importance of pressure recovery phenomenon.

3.2.1 Peak velocity, gradient and VTI

The velocity resemble those of mild native aortic valve stenosis with a maximal velocity usually >2m/s. The shape of the velocity contour is triangular with occurrence of the maximal velocity in early systole. A different pattern of the flow velocity indicates the presence of valve dysfunction. A higher gradient than 3m/sec should prompt further investigations.

The VTI is the contour of the velocity through the valve and is a qualitative but valuable index. It is difficult as previously mentioned, to differentiate high flow status from obstruction from mismatch. Other indices are than used.

3.2.2 Effective orifice area

The aortic EOA is derived with the stroke volume at the LVO, according to the continuity equation. This equation shows that in a closed hydraulic system flow is the same at different points in the system:

$$EOA_{PrAV}= CSA_{LVO}xVTI_{LVO}/VTI_{PrAV} \quad (2)$$

CSA_{LVO} is the cross sectional area of the outflow tract just underneath the valve from the parastenal long axis view, assuming a circular geometry. Attention should be given to the measure. An error will be amplified by the fact that the radius derived of this measure is used in square.

The VTI_{LVO} is the VTI proximal to the valve using pulsed wave Doppler. The sample should be located 0,5 to 1 cm below the sewing ring to avoid subvalvular acceleration.

The VTI_{PrAV} is the VTI across the valve (PrVA: Prosthetic Aortic Valve) using continuous wave Doppler.

The calculated EOA is dependant of the valve size and should therefore be compared to the effective EOA available from in vivo measurements for each type and size of valve also called projected EOA.

If calculated EOA is different of 1DSA of the EOA, it is suggestive of dysfunction of the prosthesis.

3.2.3 Doppler velocity index

The Doppler Velocity Index (DVI) is the ratio of velocity proximal to the valve (V_{LVO}) and in the valve (V_{PrAV}). It is independent of the size of the LVO and the valve. It can be approximated by the ratio of the respective peak velocities.

$$DVI=V_{LVO}/V_{PrAV} \quad (3)$$

DVI is always less than one because flow always accelerates through the valve. If it is < 0,25 it highly suggestive of significant valve obstruction.

3.2.4 The pressure recovery phenomenon

The pressure recovery phenomenon should also be evaluated. The Bernouilli equation implies that conversion of pressure to velocity is reversible. When blood flows across a stenotic orifice, velocity rises and pressure drops with the lowest pressure and highest velocity at the narrowest portion of the jet. When flow widens, flow velocity diminishes and pressure increases. This is known as pressure recovery. It is always incomplete because of energy loss due to viscosity and turbulences. The amount of energy lost varies with the shape and size of the conduit, and potentially reflect the severity of the stenosis (Garcia et al., 2000). The energy lost coefficient (ELC) can be quantified by the following equation:

$$ELC = EOA x A_A / A_A - EOA \quad (4)$$

In this equation, A_A is the aortic cross-sectional area.

Pressure recovery can occur in 2 regions: downstream the valve and in the valve. Downstream the valve there is an inverse relationship between the size of aortic root and the amount of pressure recovery. The importance of the phenomenon is generally small except in aorta smaller than 3 cm where the gradient across the valve can be overestimated (Baumgartner et al., 1992, Baumgartner et al., 1999). Within the valve, in some cases (typically in bileaflet mechanical valves), due the specific design of the valve, this phenomenon occurs. The smaller orifice located centrally between the 2 leaflets may give rise to a high velocity jet corresponding in localized pressure drops that recovers one the central flow reunites with lateral flows. This high gradient can be interpreted and lead to overestimation of the gradient across the valve and underestimation of the EOA (Baumgartner et al., 1992). This is more frequent in smaller valves. Usually it is not a problem because normal gradients expected through each valve exist as for the EOA, and are reported in the literature (Zoghbi et al., 2009).

With all these data, PPM can be diagnosed. Some very clear algorithms exist in the literature guiding the clinician in his search for PPM (Pibarot and Dumesnil, 2006, Dumesnil and Pibarot, 2011, Zoghbi et al., 2009). Based on these observations, we here present in Figure 3 maybe the most accurate algorithm, used in our unit, from the Dumesnil and Pibarot observations (Dumesnil and Pibarot, 2011).

To summarise this algorithm and concentrate on mismatch, we could resume the sequence to infirm or confirm mismatch. If a high gradient is reported, calculation of the EOA should be compared to the projected EOA. If it is similar, the EOA should then be indexed to BSA. We can than grade the severity of mismatch with cut off points of 0.85 cm2/m2 for moderate mismatch and 0,65 cm2/m2 for severe mismatch bearing in mind the pressure recovery phenomenon for small aorta.

Of course one should bear in mind that PPM and prosthesis dysfunction can coexist and that evaluation can still be challenging. Other tests can help differentiating these conditions:

- Cinefluoroscopy by imaging the motion of the leaflets in mechanical valve;
- Transesophagial echocardiography to have better images of the valve including thrombus, endocarditis and leaflets;
- Computerized tomography to image pannus, calcifications and motion of the leaflets. Anatomic orifice area can be determined by CT. It is different than EOA, being too optimistic and cannot replace EOA;
- Exercise testing can be useful. Some patients are symptomatic but echocardiography is equivocal at rest. The presence of PPM or dysfunction of the valve is associated with marked increase in gradients and pulmonary artery pressure on exercise test. Although precise cut points are not available it is likely that a rise in mean gradient >15 mmHg is significant as for native valves (Pibarot et al., 1999). Stress test can be particularly helpful in elderly patients who may claim to be asymptomatic by self limitation.

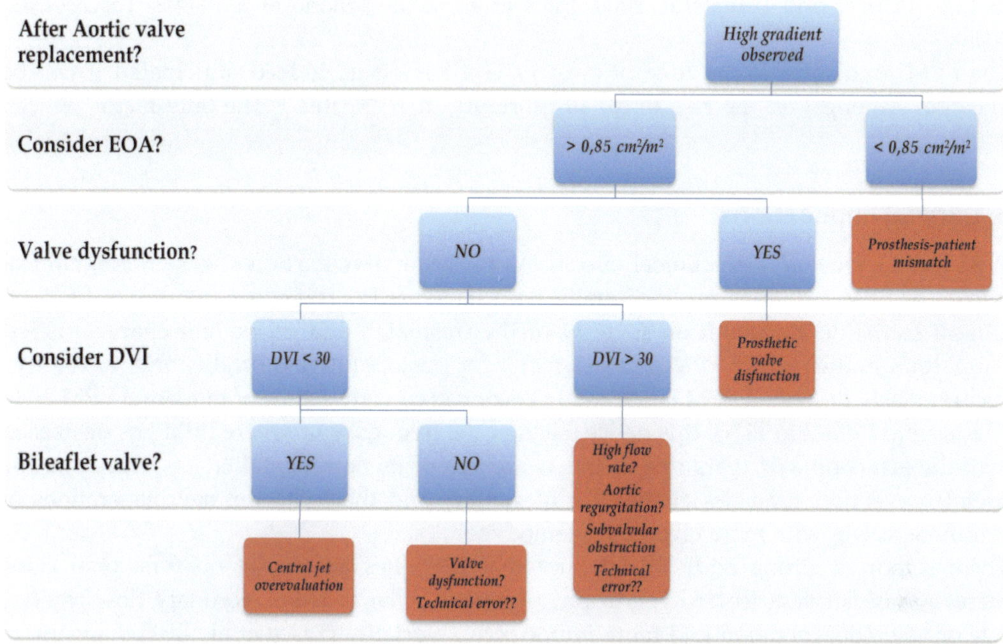

Fig. 3. Decisional algorithm to identify the origin of a abnormally hight transvalvular gradient.

4. Prediction of PPM

As previously said PPM can be estimated or predicted by using the projected EOA available for each valve type and size.

The predicted EOA measures coming from in vivo studies are well correlated with postoperative gradients and clinical outcomes (Pibarot and Dumesnil, 2006, Blackstone et al., 2003, Dumesnil and Pibarot, 2006, Koch et al., 2005).

At this stage it is important to point out that the indexed EOA derived from in vivo postoperative measures is the only parameter valid to predict PPM and postoperative gradients (Dumesnil and Pibarot, 2011, Zoghbi et al., 2009). It is thus the only one to be used.

The indexed geometric orifice area (GOA) a static manufacturing measure based on ex vivo measurements is considerably different than the iEOA. The way it is measured varies from one type of prosthesis to the other, it always overestimates the EOA being too optimistic. For similar values on indexed GOA, peak and mean gradients can double between pericardial valves and homograft's (Koch et al., 2005).

The same issue is raised by the EOA measured in vitro by manufacturers. It is also always too optimistic and overestimates the EOA derived from in vivo measurements.

Both GOA and in vitro indexes correlate poorly with postoperative gradients. Within the literature some authors are still using GOA and manufacturers data. This is one of the reasons why some detrimental effects of PPM remain partly controversial till today.

Using the indexed in vivo EOA, PPM in not infrequent. Prevalence of moderate PPM varies in the literature from 20 to 70% and severe PPM prevalence is estimated between 2

to 11% (Pibarot and Dumesnil, 2000, Blais et al., 2003, Milano et al., 2002, Tasca et al., 2005).
The PPM prediction at the time of surgery is a key issue. Indeed anticipated it can be avoided. Amongst all the risk factor of mortality in AVR, this is the only factor we can avoid.

5. Clinical implications

PPM has various adverse clinical effects. As for the native aortic valve stenosis, clinical impact of PPM increases proportionally with its severity. The consequences of PPM on clinical status depend both on severity of the mismatch and on patient characteristics. Numerous studies report PPM as a risk factor for postoperative mortality and morbidity. As previously described PPM is not rarely encountered (prevalence of moderate PPM 20 to 70%, severe PPM 2 to 11%). It is noticeable that the frequency of severe PPM has decreased over the last couple of years due to the awareness of its detrimental effects, thanks to the useful prevention strategies at the time of surgery and thanks to the new generations of prosthetic valves with more favorable haemodynamics.
There is now a strong body of evidence that PPM has an impact on functional class, regression of left ventricular hypertrophy, left ventricular function, coronary flow reserve, rate of valve degeneration and more importantly, mortality (Tasca et al., 2005, Flameng et al., 2010). Over time it has become clear that the impact of PPM depends greatly on the clinical condition of the patients.

5.1 Mortality

Considering the most important outcome, mortality, we have to distinguish early and late mortality. The impact of PPM on early mortality is more important than on late mortality given that the left ventricle is more vulnerable during early postoperative period to any hemodynamic burden imposed. Early mortality is significantly increased if PPM is severe or if moderate PPM is associated with left ventricular dysfunction (left ventricular ejection fraction (LVEF) < 40%) (Blais et al., 2003, Pibarot and Dumesnil, 2006, Urso et al., 2009). Blais et al showed in a study in 1265 patients undergoing AVR that mortality was 5% in patients with moderate PPM and normal left ventricular function, was 16% in patients with moderate PPM and depressed left ventricular function and was 67% if PPM was severe and combined with left ventricular dysfunction (Blais et al., 2003).
There are still controversies regarding late mortality. Several studies reported that PPM is an independent factor of mortality after AVR (Blais et al., 2003, Tasca et al., 2006), other concluded that PPM did not affect mortality (Blackstone et al., 2003, Koch et al., 2005). The different conclusions may result from the heterogenous populations that have been studied and the way to predict PPM (GOA or in vitro EOA). Indeed PPM clinical relevance varies with the patient characteristics. Mohty et al summarizes the impacts of PPM on late mortality in different subgroups of patients: moderate PPM increases mortality if left ventricular function is reduced (LVEF <50%) but not with normal ventricular function. Severe PPM increases mortality in patients younger than 70 years old, with a reduced left ventricular function or BMI < 30 Kg/m^2 (Mohty et al., 2009).

Blackstone and Howell have used different parameters to define mismatch (GOA, in vitro EOA). Blakstone in a very large study showed no effect of PPM on mortality but population characteristic is not well defined (Blackstone et al., 2003).

Some other studies demonstrated that PPM has no impact on mortality in the elderly (Monin et al., 2007). The relationship between age and PPM can be explained by the cardiac index requirement varying with age. Indeed younger people are more active and have a higher basal metabolic state compared with older patients. Another potential explanation is the longer exposure to PPM for the younger patients. Finally if we consider patients implanted with a bioprosthetic valve, the deterioration of the valve is likely to appear faster in younger people who are more prone to calcifications. These patients will have less "EOA reserve" if PPM is present. Higher gradient and stenosis will tend to develop faster with the combination of degeneration and PPM (Flameng et al., 2010).

Interaction between PPM and BMI should be emphasized. PPM impact on patients with a BMI< 30 kg/m2 reflects more probably that EOA should not be indexed with BSA but with a fat-free index in these obese patients. iEOA overestimates the prevalence and severity of PPM in this subgroup of patients.

Logically patients with reduced left ventricular function will not tolerate the increased burden secondary to PPM regardless of its severity (Blais et al., 2003, Kulik et al., 2006, Ruel et al., 2006).

5.2 Left ventricular hypertrophy, function and coronary flow reserve

PPM has also an impact on the left ventricle. Controversies remain about the role of PPM on the regression of the left ventricular hypertrophy. After relief of the stenosis, reduction of the left ventricular hypertrophy will occur whatsoever and the impact of the PPM on the degree of regression of left ventricular mass remains unknown. It is know recognized that the presence of systemic hypertension, metabolic syndrome, decreased vascular compliance results in an increase of the afterload of the ventricle that will not be relieved after surgery. The degree of muscular hypertrophy and interstitial fibrosis (which is not reversible) does not depend only on residual gradient: left ventricular hypertrophy regression is multifactorial and not only related to PPM.

As described earlier PPM has a significant impact on mortality if present with concomitant left ventricular dysfunction. The improvement of LV function is correlated with the increased EOA after surgery. This has been shown for surgery but also for percutaneously implanted aortic valve. Indeed recently LV function has been compared in patients surgically implanted and percutaneously implanted. LV function improved faster after transcatheter implantation mainly to the larger iEOA observed after transcatheter implantation leading to smaller gradient and better haemodynamic (Jilaihawi et al., 2010, Clavel et al., 2009).

One of the main goals of aortic valve replacement is restoration of the myocardial reserve. A persistent significant gradient across the valve affects coronary reserve recovery. Independently of the regression of the left ventricular mass, postoperative coronary vasodilatory reserve varies proportionally to the iEOA and thus to PPM (Rajappan et al., 2003).

5.3 Miscelaneous

PPM is also associated with a number of other adverse outcomes with variable clinical importance: reduced quality of life, reduced exercise capacity (Bleiziffer et al., 2008), more important residual mitral regurgitation (Unger et al., 2010), the risk of early degeneration of bioprosthetic valve with stenotic lesions (Flameng et al., 2010) and increased risk of hemorrhagic complication due to the acquired abnormalities of the Von Willebrand factor (Vincentelli et al., 2003).

6. Prevention of patient-prosthesis mismatch

Aortic valve replacement has become a simple and safe procedure through the time. Nowadays, this procedure can be accomplished with a low mortality and morbidity rate. However, there is no zero risk aortic valve replacement surgery nowadays. In this particular setting, it appears that patient-prosthesis mismatch emerges as a prominent risk factor for postoperative mortality and morbidity, and one of the few that can be acted upon. A strategy of prevention of PPM is thus of the upmost importance. Severe PPM (EOA<0,65 cm^2/m^2) must be avoided in all patients. Moderate PPM only justifies an aggressive prevention strategy in the most susceptible patients:

1. Patients younger than 65 years of age;
2. Athletes;
3. Patients with preexistent systolic dysfunction of the left ventricle with left ventricular ejection fraction less than 40%;
4. Patients with severe left ventricular muscle hypertrophy.

To the contrary, moderate PPM could be neglected in low exposed patients including:

1. Obese patient where the cardiac output is not directly proportional to the BSA;
2. Older patients.

The EOA of the prosthesis to be implanted must thus be more than 0,85 cm^2/m^2 (compilation of the body surface area of the patients is prerequired).

6.1 The choice of the prosthesis

Compared to a bioprosthesis, mechanical valves present a better EOA at the same prosthesis size. Intraoperatively, it is important to consider the EOA of the prosthesis that can fit the aortic root. A type of prosthesis with the largest EOA for a given nominal diameter should be chosen. Not all available models of prostheses for a given aortic root configuration have the same size: a size 23 model of one manufacturer may fit the same aortic root configuration as a size 21 model of another. Stentless bioprostheses claim better hemodynamic parameters than their stented counterparts. Also, recent generation bileaflet mechanical prostheses offer better EOA for a given nominal external diameter. On Table 2 and Table 3, the EOA and iEOA of o bioprosthesis and a mechanical valve are reported. We can see that mechanical valves presents better hemodynamic parameters than bioprosthesis.

6.2 The surgical technique

Surgical implantation technique also allows implantation of a larger prosthesis. The simplest way to achieve this goal is to choose a supraannular rather than annular technique (Fig. 4).

	Carpentier-Edwards Perimount®					
Prosthesis size	**19**	**21**	**23**	**25**	**27**	**29**
EOA (cm²/m²)	1,1	1,3	1,5	1,8	1,8	
BSA (m²)						
1	1,10	1,30	1,50	1,80	1,80	
1,1	1,00	1,18	1,36	1,64	1,64	
1,2	0,92	1,08	1,25	1,50	1,50	
1,3	0,85	1,00	1,15	1,38	1,38	
1,4	0,79	93,00	1,07	1,38	1,38	
1,5	0,73	0,87	1,00	1,20	1,20	
1,6	0,69	0,81	0,94	1,12	1,12	
1,7	0,65	0,76	0,88	1,06	1,06	
1,8	0,61	0,72	0,83	1,00	1,00	
1,9	0,58	0,68	0,79	0,95	0,95	
2	0,55	0,65	0,75	0,90	0,90	
2,1	0,52	0,62	0,71	0,86	0,86	
2,2	0,50	0,59	0,68	0,82	0,82	
2,3	0,48	0,56	0,65	0,78	0,78	
2,4	0,46	0,54	0,62	0,75	0,75	
2,5	0,44	0,52	0,60	0,72	0,72	

Table 2. Eoa and iEOA of a performant bioprosthesis (Blais et al., 2003).

	St Jude Medical Regent®					
Prosthesis size	**19**	**21**	**23**	**25**	**27**	**29**
EOA (cm²/m²)	1,5	2	2,4	2,5	3,6	4,8
BSA (m²)						
1	1,50	2,00	2,40	2,50	3,60	4,80
1,1	1,36	1,82	2,18	2,27	3,27	4,36
1,2	1,25	1,67	2,00	2,08	3,00	4,00
1,3	1,15	1,54	1,85	1,92	2,77	3,69
1,4	1,07	1,43	1,71	1,78	2,57	3,43
1,5	1,00	1,33	1,60	1,67	2,40	3,20
1,6	0,94	1,25	1,50	1,56	2,25	3,00
1,7	0,88	1,18	1,41	1,47	2,12	2,82
1,8	0,83	1,11	1,33	1,39	2,00	2,67
1,9	0,79	1,05	1,26	1,32	1,89	2,53
2	0,75	1,00	1,20	1,25	1,80	2,40
2,1	0,71	0,95	1,14	1,16	1,71	2,29
2,2	0,68	0,91	1,09	1,14	1,64	2,18
2,3	0,65	0,87	1,04	1,09	1,56	2,09
2,4	0,62	0,83	1,00	1,04	1,50	2,00
2,5	0,60	0,80	0,96	1,00	1,44	1,92

Table 3. Eoa and iEOA of a performant bileaflet mechanical valve (Blais et al., 2003).

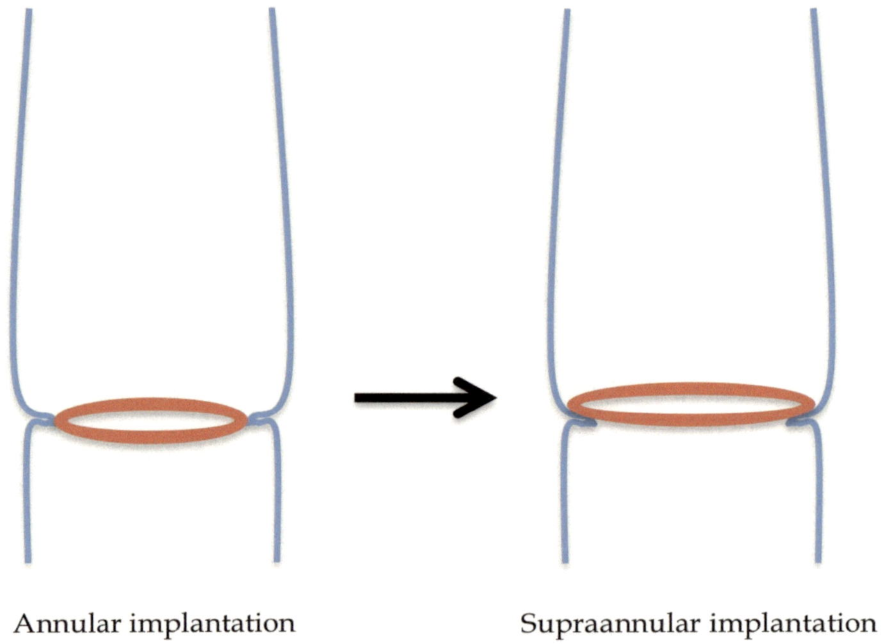

Fig. 4. Illustration of the benefit to implant the prosthesis in a supraannular technique.

A more aggressive, and more potentially beneficial technique, consist to associate aortic valve replacement and enlargement of the aortic root and annulus. The Manouguian technique inserts a widening patch in the left-non coronary commissure and allows implantation of a prosthesis one to two sizes larger (Manouguian and Seybold-Epting, 1979). Unfortunately, the presence of important aortic root calcifications limits the application of this technique. Briefly, an oblique aortotomy is performed and aimed to descend at the left-non coronary sinus, through the aorto-mitral transition (Figure 5).

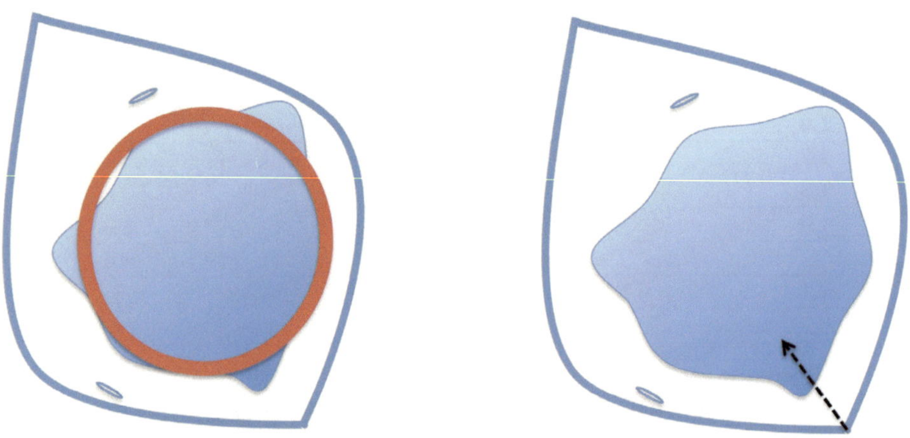

Fig. 5. Illustration of the transannular incision realized in the Manouguian technique.

A widening patch is then implanted to close this incision (Figure 6) and the prosthesis is thereafter sutured to the aortic annulus and to the reconstructive patch (Figure 7).

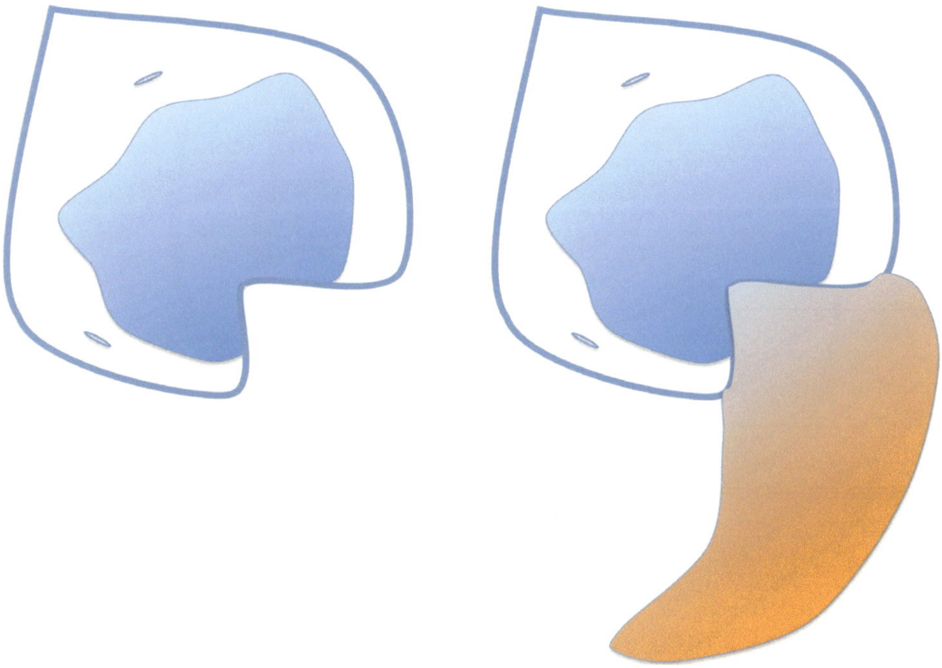

Fig. 6. Illustration of the enlarging patch reconstruction of the incision.

The Figure 7 shows the significant oversizing allowed by the technique compare to the initial prosthesis size matched to the initial annulus. The aortotomy is closed with the enlargement patch after the implantation of the aortic valve prosthesis.

During this procedure, the incision in the aortoventricular membrane must be carefully performed and not extended to deep in the mitral annulus, the anterior mitral leaflet and the left atrium. The reconstruction patch may in this particular setting interfere with the hinging portion of the anterior mitral leaflet.

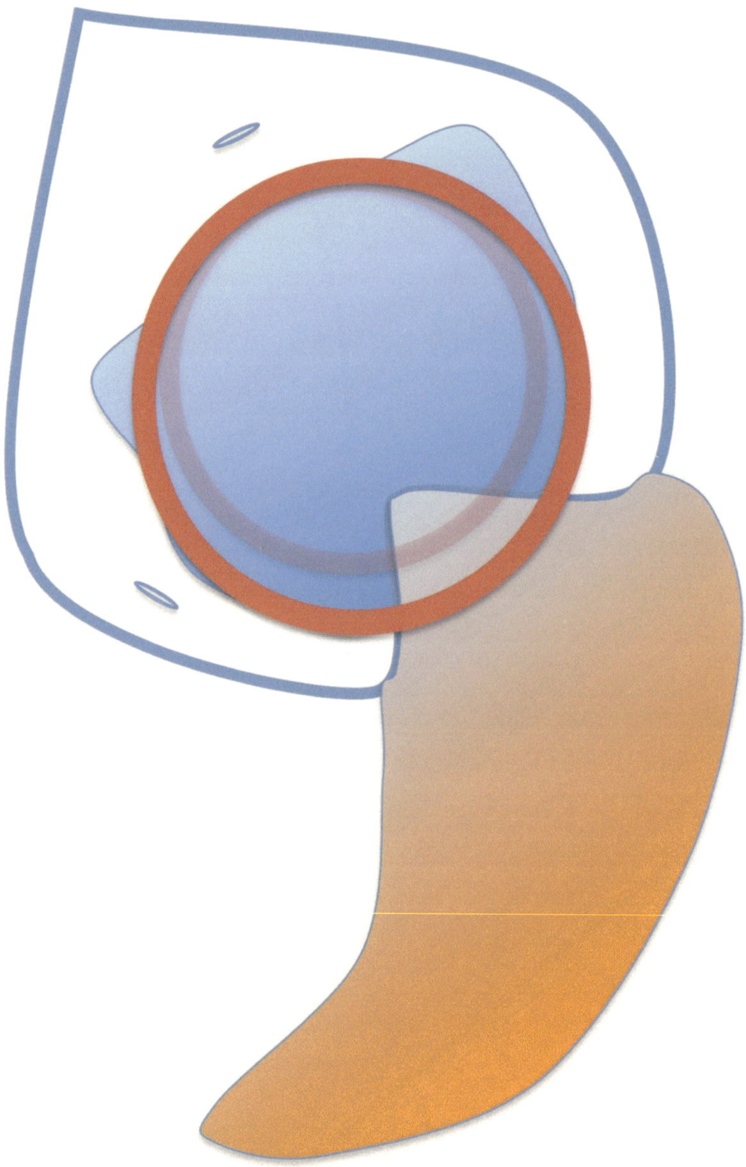

Fig. 7. Illustration of the realized oversizing allowed by the Manouguian technique.

The overall surgical strategy that we proposed is illustrated in the Figure 8. The first possibility to match the implanted valve to the patient is to realize a supraannular implantation. If this surgical technique is insufficient, we should consider an alternative second choice in the prosthesis strategy, ie a bileaflet new generation of mechanical prosthesis (an old patient with atrial fibrillation...). The last possibility is to realize a Manouguian enlargement of the aortic annulus, if possible.

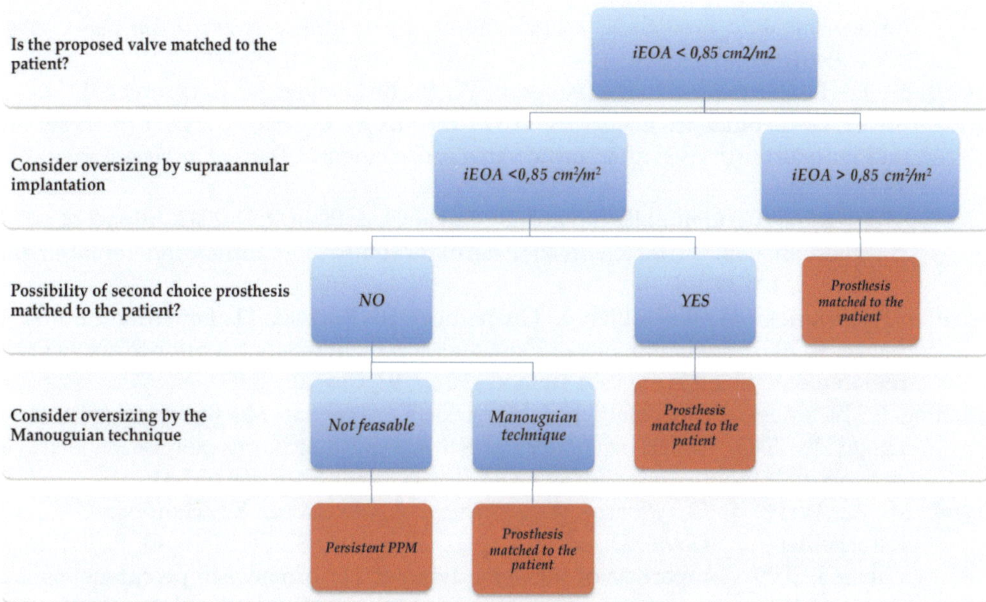

Fig. 8. Surgical strategy to avoid a patient-prosthesis mismatch.

It should be mentioned that some patients present with a hypoplastic aorto-ventricular junction. Most of them are referred to surgery during childhood. In such situation, a radical enlargement of both the aortic valve annulus and the left ventricular outflow tract should be performed. The anterior technique, first described by Konno in 1974 (Konno et al., 1975), consists in a wide opening of the aortic valve annulus and of the interventricular septum with an oblique incision at 5mm to the left side of the right coronary ostium. This technique is far more complex than the Manouguian technique and may lead to severe complications, particularly an iatrogenic ventricular septal defect or atrioventricular block.

7. Conclusions

Patient-prosthesis mismatch is probably the most frequently encountered hemodynamic problem after aortic valve replacement. All the patients are not equally exposed to this problem and clinical consequences may be variable from one to another. However, the consequences may lead to an increased mortality and worsen symptomatic improvements after the aortic valve replacement. Though, prevention of this mechanism is the key point in symptomatic patients that should be operated on. Indexed EOA of the implanted valve should be systematically calculated from reference values of the EOA of the prosthesis, and surgical strategies adapted to allow implantation of prosthesis with iEOA matched to the patient.

8. References

Baumgartner, H., Khan, S., DeRobertis, M., Czer, L. & Maurer, G. 1992. Effect of prosthetic aortic valve design on the Doppler-catheter gradient correlation: an in vitro study of normal St. Jude, Medtronic-Hall, Starr-Edwards and Hancock valves. *J Am Coll Cardiol*, 19, 324-32.

Baumgartner, H., Stefenelli, T., Niederberger, J., Schima, H. & Maurer, G. 1999. "Overestimation" of catheter gradients by Doppler ultrasound in patients with aortic stenosis: a predictable manifestation of pressure recovery. *J Am Coll Cardiol*, 33, 1655-61.

Blackstone, E. H., Cosgrove, D. M., Jamieson, W. R., Birkmeyer, N. J., Lemmer, J. H., Jr., Miller, D. C., Butchart, E. G., Rizzoli, G., Yacoub, M. & Chai, A. 2003. Prosthesis size and long-term survival after aortic valve replacement. *J Thorac Cardiovasc Surg*, 126, 783-96.

Blais, C., Dumesnil, J. G., Baillot, R., Simard, S., Doyle, D. & Pibarot, P. 2003. Impact of valve prosthesis-patient mismatch on short-term mortality after aortic valve replacement. *Circulation*, 108, 983-8.

Bleiziffer, S., Eichinger, W. B., Hettich, I., Guenzinger, R., Ruzicka, D., Bauernschmitt, R. & Lange, R. 2007. Prediction of valve prosthesis-patient mismatch prior to aortic valve replacement: which is the best method? *Heart*, 93, 615-20.

Bleiziffer, S., Eichinger, W. B., Hettich, I., Ruzicka, D., Wottke, M., Bauernschmitt, R. & Lange, R. 2008. Impact of patient-prosthesis mismatch on exercise capacity in patients after bioprosthetic aortic valve replacement. *Heart*, 94, 637-41.

Clavel, M. A., Webb, J. G., Pibarot, P., Altwegg, L., Dumont, E., Thompson, C., De Larochelliere, R., Doyle, D., Masson, J. B., Bergeron, S., Bertrand, O. F. & Rodes-Cabau, J. 2009. Comparison of the hemodynamic performance of percutaneous and surgical bioprostheses for the treatment of severe aortic stenosis. *J Am Coll Cardiol*, 53, 1883-91.

Dumesnil, J. G. & Pibarot, P. 2006. Prosthesis-patient mismatch and clinical outcomes: the evidence continues to accumulate. *J Thorac Cardiovasc Surg*, 131, 952-5.

Dumesnil, J. G. & Pibarot, P. 2011. Prosthesis-Patient Mismatch: An Update. *Curr Cardiol Rep*.

Flameng, W., Herregods, M. C., Vercalsteren, M., Herijgers, P., Bogaerts, K. & Meuris, B. 2010. Prosthesis-patient mismatch predicts structural valve degeneration in bioprosthetic heart valves. *Circulation*, 121, 2123-9.

Garcia, D., Pibarot, P., Dumesnil, J. G., Sakr, F. & Durand, L. G. 2000. Assessment of aortic valve stenosis severity: A new index based on the energy loss concept. *Circulation*, 101, 765-71.

Jilaihawi, H., Chin, D., Spyt, T., Jeilan, M., Vasa-Nicotera, M., Bence, J., Logtens, E. & Kovac, J. 2010. Prosthesis-patient mismatch after transcatheter aortic valve implantation with the Medtronic-Corevalve bioprosthesis. *Eur Heart J*, 31, 857-64.

Koch, C. G., Khandwala, F., Estafanous, F. G., Loop, F. D. & Blackstone, E. H. 2005. Impact of prosthesis-patient size on functional recovery after aortic valve replacement. *Circulation*, 111, 3221-9.

Konno, S., Imai, Y., Iida, Y., Nakajima, M. & Tatsuno, K. 1975. A new method for prosthetic valve replacement in congenital aortic stenosis associated with hypoplasia of the aortic valve ring. *J Thorac Cardiovasc Surg*, 70, 909-17.

Kulik, A., Burwash, I. G., Kapila, V., Mesana, T. G. & Ruel, M. 2006. Long-term outcomes after valve replacement for low-gradient aortic stenosis: impact of prosthesis-patient mismatch. *Circulation,* 114, I553-8.

Manouguian, S. & Seybold-Epting, W. 1979. Patch enlargement of the aortic valve ring by extending the aortic incision into the anterior mitral leaflet. New operative technique. *J Thorac Cardiovasc Surg,* 78, 402-12.

Milano, A. D., De Carlo, M., Mecozzi, G., D'Alfonso, A., Scioti, G., Nardi, C. & Bortolotti, U. 2002. Clinical outcome in patients with 19-mm and 21-mm St. Jude aortic prostheses: comparison at long-term follow-up. *Ann Thorac Surg,* 73, 37-43.

Mohty, D., Dumesnil, J. G., Echahidi, N., Mathieu, P., Dagenais, F., Voisine, P. & Pibarot, P. 2009. Impact of prosthesis-patient mismatch on long-term survival after aortic valve replacement: influence of age, obesity, and left ventricular dysfunction. *J Am Coll Cardiol,* 53, 39-47.

Monin, J. L., Monchi, M., Kirsch, M. E., Petit-Eisenmann, H., Baleynaud, S., Chauvel, C., Metz, D., Adams, C., Quere, J. P., Gueret, P. & Tribouilloy, C. 2007. Low-gradient aortic stenosis: impact of prosthesis-patient mismatch on survival. *Eur Heart J,* 28, 2620-6.

Pibarot, P. & Dumesnil, J. G. 2000. Hemodynamic and clinical impact of prosthesis-patient mismatch in the aortic valve position and its prevention. *J Am Coll Cardiol,* 36, 1131-41.

Pibarot, P. & Dumesnil, J. G. 2006. Prosthesis-patient mismatch: definition, clinical impact, and prevention. *Heart,* 92, 1022-9.

Pibarot, P., Dumesnil, J. G., Briand, M., Laforest, I. & Cartier, P. 2000. Hemodynamic performance during maximum exercise in adult patients with the ross operation and comparison with normal controls and patients with aortic bioprostheses. *Am J Cardiol,* 86, 982-8.

Pibarot, P., Dumesnil, J. G., Jobin, J., Cartier, P., Honos, G. & Durand, L. G. 1999. Hemodynamic and physical performance during maximal exercise in patients with an aortic bioprosthetic valve: comparison of stentless versus stented bioprostheses. *J Am Coll Cardiol,* 34, 1609-17.

Rahimtoola, S. H. 1978. The problem of valve prosthesis-patient mismatch. *Circulation,* 58, 20-4.

Rajappan, K., Rimoldi, O. E., Camici, P. G., Bellenger, N. G., Pennell, D. J. & Sheridan, D. J. 2003. Functional changes in coronary microcirculation after valve replacement in patients with aortic stenosis. *Circulation,* 107, 3170-5.

Ruel, M., Al-Faleh, H., Kulik, A., Chan, K. L., Mesana, T. G. & Burwash, I. G. 2006. Prosthesis-patient mismatch after aortic valve replacement predominantly affects patients with preexisting left ventricular dysfunction: effect on survival, freedom from heart failure, and left ventricular mass regression. *J Thorac Cardiovasc Surg,* 131, 1036-44.

Ruel, M., Rubens, F. D., Masters, R. G., Pipe, A. L., Bedard, P., Hendry, P. J., Lam, B. K., Burwash, I. G., Goldstein, W. G., Brais, M. P., Keon, W. J. & Mesana, T. G. 2004. Late incidence and predictors of persistent or recurrent heart failure in patients with aortic prosthetic valves. *J Thorac Cardiovasc Surg,* 127, 149-59.

Tasca, G., Brunelli, F., Cirillo, M., DallaTomba, M., Mhagna, Z., Troise, G. & Quaini, E. 2005. Impact of valve prosthesis-patient mismatch on left ventricular mass regression following aortic valve replacement. *Ann Thorac Surg*, 79, 505-10.

Tasca, G., Mhagna, Z., Perotti, S., Centurini, P. B., Sabatini, T., Amaducci, A., Brunelli, F., Cirillo, M., Dalla Tomba, M., Quaini, E., Troise, G. & Pibarot, P. 2006. Impact of prosthesis-patient mismatch on cardiac events and midterm mortality after aortic valve replacement in patients with pure aortic stenosis. *Circulation*, 113, 570-6.

Unger, P., Dedobbeleer, C., Van Camp, G., Plein, D., Cosyns, B. & Lancellotti, P. 2010. Mitral regurgitation in patients with aortic stenosis undergoing valve replacement. *Heart*, 96, 9-14.

Urso, S., Sadaba, R. & Aldamiz-Echevarria, G. 2009. Is patient-prosthesis mismatch an independent risk factor for early and mid-term overall mortality in adult patients undergoing aortic valve replacement? *Interact Cardiovasc Thorac Surg*, 9, 510-8.

Vincentelli, A., Susen, S., Le Tourneau, T., Six, I., Fabre, O., Juthier, F., Bauters, A., Decoene, C., Goudemand, J., Prat, A. & Jude, B. 2003. Acquired von Willebrand syndrome in aortic stenosis. *N Engl J Med*, 349, 343-9.

Zoghbi, W. A., Chambers, J. B., Dumesnil, J. G., Foster, E., Gottdiener, J. S., Grayburn, P. A., Khandheria, B. K., Levine, R. A., Marx, G. R., Miller, F. A., Jr., Nakatani, S., Quinones, M. A., Rakowski, H., Rodriguez, L. L., Swaminathan, M., Waggoner, A. D., *et al.* 2009. Recommendations for evaluation of prosthetic valves with echocardiography and doppler ultrasound: a report From the American Society of Echocardiography's Guidelines and Standards Committee and the Task Force on Prosthetic Valves, developed in conjunction with the American College of Cardiology Cardiovascular Imaging Committee, Cardiac Imaging Committee of the American Heart Association, the European Association of Echocardiography, a registered branch of the European Society of Cardiology, the Japanese Society of Echocardiography and the Canadian Society of Echocardiography, endorsed by the American College of Cardiology Foundation, American Heart Association, European Association of Echocardiography, a registered branch of the European Society of Cardiology, the Japanese Society of Echocardiography, and Canadian Society of Echocardiography. *J Am Soc Echocardiogr*, 22, 975-1014; quiz 1082-4.

6

Pharmacologic and Non-Pharmacologic Treatment of Chronic Atrial Fibrillation – With Special Reference to Valvular Atrial Fibrillation in Rheumatic Heart Disease

Mohan Nair, Sanjeeb Patra and Vanita Arora
Max healthcare Superspeciality Hospital, New Delhi
India

1. Introduction

Atrial fibrillation (AF), the most commonly encountered arrhythmia in clinical practice, is associated with significant morbidity and mortality. Of great significance are heart failure and stroke.[1] With increased incidence and prevalence of AF, it represents a growing clinical and economic burden. AF is also a progressive disease secondary to continuous structural remodeling of the atria because of AF itself, to changes associated with ageing and to deterioration of underlying heart disease. Current management aims at preventing the recurrence of AF and its consequences and includes risk assessment and prevention of stroke, control of ventricular rate and rhythm control therapies including antiarrhythmic drugs and catheter or surgical ablation.

2. Classification

The nomenclature used to classify AF has been diverse. AF can be acute (first detectable episode whether symptomatic or not) or chronic (paroxysmal, persistent, and long-standing persistent), or finally permanent. According to a consensus document[2], paroxysmal AF is defined as at least two episodes that terminate spontaneously within 7 days. Persistent AF is defined as lasting more than 7 days, or lasting less than 7 days but necessitating pharmacologic or electrical cardio version. Permanent AF is defined as lasting more than 1 year.
These definitions apply only to episodes that last at least 30 seconds and have no identifiable reversible cause, such as acute pulmonary disease or hyperthyroidism. Both paroxysmal and persistent atrial fibrillations are potentially recurrent arrhythmias. Paroxysmal atrial fibrillation may become persistent with time; and both paroxysmal and persistent AF may become permanent.
The term "lone atrial fibrillation" refers to AF in young people (aged under 60) in whom no apparent cause can be identified.

3. Pathophysiology

The exact mechanisms by which cardiovascular risk factors predispose to AF are not understood fully but are under intense investigation. Catecholamine excess, hemodynamic stress, atrial ischemia, atrial inflammation, metabolic stress, and neurohumoral cascade activation are all purported to promote AF. Although the precise mechanisms that cause AF are incompletely understood, AF appears to require both an initiating event and a permissive atrial substrate. AF results from multiple re-entrant electrical wavelets that move randomly around the atria. These wavelets are initiated by electrical triggers, commonly located in the myocardial sleeves extending from the left atrium to the proximal 5-6 cm portions of the pulmonary veins[3]. Other sites in the left and right atria and in the proximal superior vena cava may less frequently trigger atrial fibrillation[4, 5]. Once triggered, the atrial tissue harbors these wavelets and promotes re-entry, thus facilitating persistence of the arrhythmia. A period of AF initially induces electrophysiological changes ("electrical remodeling") followed by structural changes ("structural remodeling"), which facilitate its persistence- hence the phrase "atrial fibrillation begets atrial fibrillation"[6, 7].

Common causes of Atrial Fibrillation	
Cardiovascular	Non-cardiovasular
• Rheumatic heart disease • Hypertension • Coronary artery disease • Congestive heart failure • Non rheumatic valvular heart disease • Sick sinus syndrome • Wolf-Parkinson-white syndrome • Pericarditis • Endocarditis • Cardiomyopathy • Congenital heart disease	• Endocrine disorders (e.g.,Hyperthyroidism) • Respiratory causes (e.g., pneumonia, pulmonary thromboembolism) • Alcohol and drug use

Atrial fibrillation with poor ventricular rate control can cause electrical and structural remodeling of the ventricle, leading to ventricular dilatation and impairment of systolic function, known as "tachycardia induced cardiomyopathy".

Stroke and thromboembolism are a major cause of mortality and morbidity associated with AF, and the underlying pathophysiological basis of this is a prothrombotic or hypercoagulable state, in association with abnormalities of blood flow (atrial stasis, for example) and endothelial or endocardial damage.

The concept of primary prevention of AF with interventions targeting the development of substrate and modifying risk factors for AF has emerged as a result of recent experiments that suggested novel targets for mechanism-based therapies.

Upstream therapy refers to the use of non-antiarrhythmic drugs that modify the atrial substrate- or target-specific mechanisms of AF to prevent the occurrence or recurrence of the arrhythmia. Angiotensin converting enzyme inhibitors (ACEIs) and angiotensin receptor blockers (ARBs) may be effective in AF prevention in patients with hypertension, left ventricular hypertrophy, and congestive heart failure, as well as in post myocardial infarction patients with depressed left ventricular function[8]. Also statins and omega-3 polyunsaturated fatty acids, and possibly corticosteroids. Animal experiments have compellingly demonstrated the protective effect of these agents against electrical and structural atrial remodeling in association with AF. The key targets of upstream therapy are structural changes in the atria, such as fibrosis, hypertrophy, inflammation, and oxidative stress, but direct and indirect effects on atrial ion channels, gap junctions, and calcium handling are also applied. Although there have been no formal randomized controlled studies (RCTs) in the primary prevention setting, retrospective analyses and reports from the studies in which AF was a pre-specified secondary endpoint have shown a sustained reduction in new-onset AF with ACEIs and ARBs in patients with significant underlying heart disease (e.g. left ventricular dysfunction and hypertrophy), and in the incidence of AF after cardiac surgery in patients treated with statins.

4. Management of AF

AF management creates a high economic burden because of the concomitant presence of heart failure, coronary artery disease, hypertension, and the need for frequent hospitalizations. Expensive antiarrhythmic drugs and interventional procedures are other important factors that raise the costs of AF care.

Four major aspects should be considered in the AF management[9]:

i. Symptom control by slowing ventricular response during paroxysmal or persistent AF and long-term rate control in permanent AF
ii. Cardioversion to sinus rhythm
iii. Maintenance of sinus rhythm after successful cardioversion
iv. Prevention of complications and thromboembolic events.

Rhythm versus Rate Control

In order to prevent the complications and symptoms of AF two main strategies exist.

1. Rhythm control: converting the patient's rhythm to sinus and maintaining the sinus rhythm.
2. Rate control: slowing the ventricular response rate without insisting on conversion to sinus rhythm.

The initial therapy after onset of AF should always include adequate antithrombotic treatment and control of the ventricular rate. The goal is to control the ventricular rate adequately whenever recurrent AF occurs.

From a theoretical point of view, converting AF into sinus rhythm is the best option. Nonetheless; the most important trials reported in the existing literature thus far have mentioned no significant difference in terms of quality of life and other outcomes between the two strategies. It seems that the side effects of antiarrhythmic agents (pro-arrhythmia) in the long term, poor efficacy of drugs in the maintenance of sinus rhythm, and inappropriate discontinuation of anticoagulants in the patients who still have AF episodes can interfere with good results in the rhythm-control arm[27]. Therefore, many experts believe that rhythm control with safe antiarrhythmic drugs or catheter ablation will play an important role in the AF management.

The main agents for slowing ventricular response in AF are beta blockers, calcium channel blockers, and digoxin[28]. Beta-blockers and calcium channel blockers are first-line agents for rate control in atrial fibrillation. These drugs can be administered either intravenously or orally. They are effective at rest and with exertion. Caution should be exercised in patients with reactive airway disease who are given beta-blockers. Digoxin is sometimes used in the acute setting but does little to control the ventricular rate in active patients. As such, it is rarely used as mono therapy. The therapeutic window for digoxin as mono therapy for rate control is narrow and would typically yield toxic levels. Thus, there may be circumstances that this drug is used as adjunctive therapy to beta-blockers or calcium channel blockers. Caution should be exercised in elderly patients and those with renal failure receiving digoxin. Digoxin is indicated in patients with heart failure and reduced LV function.

Amiodarone has a Class IIa recommendation from the ACC/AHA/ESC for use as a rate controlling agent for patients who are intolerant of or unresponsive to other agents. Caution should be exercised in those not receiving anticoagulation as amiodarone can promote cardioversion.

Criteria for rate control vary with patient age but usually involve achieving ventricular rates between 60 and 80 bpm at rest and between 90 and 115 bpm during moderate exercise.

The potential benefits of strict (resting heart rate <80 bpm, heart rate <110 bpm during moderate exercise) versus lenient (resting heart rate 110 bpm) rate control were addressed in the RACE II trial of patients with permanent AF[29]. The RACE II study shows that lenientrate control <110 bpm is not inferior to strict-rate control <80 bpm. As lenient-rate control is generally more convenient, requiring fewer outpatient visits and examinations, lenient-rate control may be adopted as a reasonable strategy in patients with permanent AF.

In the AFFIRM study, there was no survival difference between rate-control and rhythm-control strategies. In addition, the lower risk of adverse drug effects in the rate-control arm conferred some advantages in this arm. A post-hoc analysis of the AFFIRM data proved that there was no significant benefit in the rhythm-control group versus the rate-control group in patients with AF and left ventricular dysfunction[30]. The RACE study showed that for the prevention of cardiovascular mortality and morbidity in AF, rhythm control was not superior to rate control[31]. In the PIAF trial, clinical outcomes were similar between the rate-control group and the rhythm-control group but exercise tolerance was better in the rhythm-control arm[32].

However rhythm-control strategy is more popular than the rate-control strategy worldwide. Symptom control and quality of life generally are better when sinus rhythm is restored and maintained. Treatment analysis from the AFFIRM study[42] showed that the presence of sinus rhythm was associated with a 47% reduction in mortality and that the use of AAD was associated with a significant increase in mortality of 49%, suggesting a potential benefit of sinus rhythm maintenance in a non-pharmacological manner.

We hope that with the advent of new drugs for both rhythm control and anticoagulation, maintenance of sinus rhythm after cardioversion can be a more realistic goal.

4.1 Cardioversion to sinus rhythm

As a result of atrial remodelling, the longer the duration of AF the less successful is the cardioversion. Predictors of recurrence of AF include long standing atrial fibrillation (duration greater than three months), heart failure, structural heart disease, hypertension, increasing age (over 70), and increased left atrial size[10].

Although left atrial size is related to the duration of AF, a left atrial diameter greater than 6.5 cm is associated with an increased risk of recurrence[11].

Cardioversion carries a 5-7% risk of thromboembolism without anticoagulation and a 1-2% risk after conventional anticoagulation[12]. Prolonged anticoagulation is not needed when patients present within 48 hours of onset of AF. Such patients may be safely cardioverted irrespective of whether heparin has been administered since presentation. Administration of heparin is recommended to all patients with an acute presentation, however, to allow flexibility in subsequent management of the arrhythmia[13].

For stable patients, in whom the onset of AF is uncertain or greater than 48 hours, anticoagulation for a minimum of three weeks before cardioversion is recommended, to allow resolution of potential thrombi. As atrial mechanical activity may not resume concurrently with electrical activity, anticoagulation should be continued for at least four weeks after cardioversion.

An alternative approach is to use transoesophageal echocardiography to exclude atrial thrombi before cardioversion is attempted. The presence of an atrial thrombus necessitates four to six weeks of anticoagulation before cardioversion. Even with this strategy, anticoagulation should be continued for at least four weeks after cardioversion.

4.2 Pharmacological cardioversion

Pharmacological cardioversion should be reserved for haemodynamically stable patients with symptoms. In general, class I and class III antiarrhythmic agents are commonly used for pharmacological cardio version and maintenance of sinus rhythm. In AF episodes lasting less than 48 hours cardio version rate for class IC and III drugs is approximately 60-80%[14].

In a randomised trial comparing flecainide, propafenone, and amiodarone for cardioversion of recent onset AF, conversion to sinus rhythm occurred in 90%, 72%, and 64% of patients respectively[15]. Class IC drugs (flecainide and propafenone) should be avoided in patients with underlying ischaemic heart disease or impaired left ventricular function. Amiodarone can be used in such patients, although the time to conversion can range from days to weeks.

Ibutilide is a class III antiarrhythmic agent that can convert AF to sinus rhythm more rapidly than can procainamide or sotalol. It has been shown that ibutilide has no significant advantage compared with amiodarone for the conversion of AF but severe hypotension was not seen with ibutilide[23]. For acute AF, conversion to sinus rhythm with ibutilide is about 59%, but there is 1.7% risk of polymorphic ventricular tachycardia with this drug. As a result, it is advised to keep the patients receiving ibutilide under monitoring for at least 24 hours after the infusion of this drug[24].

Dofetilide is another class III antiarrhythmic drug that can be used for maintaining sinus rhythm in congestive heart failure patients with AF. The DIAMOND CHF trial showed that it could reduce hospitalization due to heart failure. Heart failure worsening was reduced by 25%.[25]Dofetilide is known to be more effective in patients with persistent AF compared with those with paroxysmal AF, and significant proarrhythmic adverse effects can occur even with close monitoring.

Vernakalant is an atrial-selective drug treatment for atrial fibrillation which affects Na+ and several K+ channels in the heart. Vernakalant is most often used intravenously to stop recent-onset AF. A long-term oral preparation, however, is in development. Several placebo-controlled studies have shown vernakalant to be effective in eliminating AF in about 50% of patients with limited side effects[16, 17]. In these studies, vernakalant was most effective for treatment of recent-onset AF, but rarely effective at all for long-standing AF. Common side effects of vernakalant include nausea, sneezing and dysgeusia. The FDA has recommended vernakalant as an intravenous treatment for recent-onset AF.

The 'Pill-in-the-poket' approach may be used in selected, symptomatic patient with infrequent episodes of AF. Oral propafenone (450-600mg) or flecainide (200-300mg) is taken when symptoms of AF occur[18].

4.3 Electrical cardioversion

Synchronised external direct current cardioversion is a safe procedure with success rates of 70-90%[19]. It is used acutely in patients who are haemodynamically compromised or electively as an alternative to pharmacological cardioversion. Electrical cardioversion is usually done under conscious sedation. If this is unsuccessful, adjunctive antiarrhythmic treatment with class III agents such as dofetilide, sotalol, and amiodarone can help to restore sinus rhythm.

4.4 Maintenance of sinus rhythm

Class III antiarrhythmic agents have an important role as a part of cardioversion strategy and maintaining sinus rhythm. Amiodarone, which is the hallmark drug in this group and most frequently used antiarrhythmic drug for AF treatment, is a relatively safe and effective drug but frequent adverse effects like thyroid dysfunction, pulmonary fibrosis, dermatological changes, and ophthalmic involvement have been reported with its long-term use[20].

Dronedarone is a benzofuran-derivate of amiodarone with the same electropharmacological profile36 but without side effects on the pulmonary system[21]. It has a shorter half-life than amiodarone (1 - 2 days). The recommended oral dose of dronedarone is 400 mg twice a day with meals. The ANDROMEDA study was terminated prematurely because of increased mortality due to the worsening of heart failure in the dronedarone group. Therefore, dronedarone is contraindicated in patients with moderate to severe heart failure[26]. The major adverse cardiac effects of dronedarone are bradycardia and QT prolongation. Torsades de pointes have been reported[22]. Cases of rare but severe hepatic injury associated with use of dronedarone reported. Periodic monitoring of liver-function test should be done especially in the first six months of treatment.

Dronedarone was approved by the American FDA in March, 2009, for sinus-rhythm maintenance in patients with a history of atrial fibrillation/flutter with ejection fraction greater than 35%.

4.5 Reduction of thromboembolic risk

Atrial fibrillation can predispose clot formation in the left atrium and consequently ischemic stroke and extra cranial thromboembolism[33]. When stroke occurs in association with atrial fibrillation, patients have a greater mortality and morbidity, longer hospital stays, and greater disability than those without AF. If AF persists for two days, left atrium thrombosis could be seen in 5 - 14% of patients[34]. It might, subsequently, become fragmented and embolize to the peripheral atrial system[35].

Pooled data from trials comparing antithrombotic treatment with placebo have shown that warfarin reduces the risk of stroke by 62% (95% confidence interval 48% to 72%) and that aspirin alone reduces the risk by 22% (2% to 38%). Overall, in high risk patients, warfarin was better than aspirin in preventing strokes, with a relative risk reduction of 36% (48% to 72%). The risk of major haemorrhage with warfarin was twice that with aspirin[36].

Anticoagulation treatment needs to be tailored individually for patients on the basis of age, comorbidities, and contraindications. In patients with valvular heart disease or high-risk individuals (according to the $CHADS_2$ or $CHA_2DS_2VAS_C$ scoring), warfarin is the drug of choice. In low-risk conditions, aspirin can be used[37].

Oral anticoagulation therapy with warfarin proved superior to clopidogrel plus ASA for prevention of vascular events in AF patients. Treatment with clopidogrel plus ASA was associated with bleeding risk similar to treatment with warfarin[38]. In the ACTIVE-A trial, AF patients for whom oral anticoagulation with warfarin was considered unsuitable, the addition of clopidogrel to ASA reduced the risk of major vascular events, especially stroke, and increased the risk of major hemorrhage[39].

Dabigatran is a new, potent, direct and competitive inhibitor of thrombin. Its half-life is 12 to 17 hours, and it does not require regular monitoring. AF patients receiving Dabigatran 110 mg twice daily had similar rates of stroke and systemic embolism compared with those using warfarin, but with lower rates of major bleeding. At a dose of 150 mg twice daily, the rate of stroke and systemic embolism is lower but the rate of major bleeding is similar to warfarin[40].

Apixaban, a novel factor Xa inhibitor, was tested in the AVERROES trial in patients unsuitable for warfarin therapy and at increased risk of stroke. The trial was stopped prematurely because of clear benefit in favor of apixaban, compared to aspirin[41].

4.6 Non-pharmacological therapy

Many non-pharmacological treatments have been developed for the management of AF and some even afford a possible "cure".

4.7 Radiofrequency catheter ablation

The past decade has witnessed radiofrequency catheter ablation of AF evolve from an experimental procedure to an important treatment option for many patients with AF. Randomized controlled trials now confirm that left atrial ablation is superior to antiarrhythmic drug therapy in maintaining sinus rhythm over time[52-54].

Curative catheter ablation techniques initially attempted to mimic the lesions created by the surgical Maze procedure, resulting in limited success with a substantial complication rate. In 1998, Haissaguerre et al. first demonstrated that pulmonary veins (PVs) provided focal firings triggering the occurrence of paroxysmal AF[3]. They showed that as many as 94% of such triggers originated from the PVs and that the elimination of these foci by radiofrequency (RF) energy applications in the PVs could cure the paroxysmal form of AF, which became the cornerstone of curative ablation of AF. However, it turned out that high recurrence rates of AF and late development of PV stenosis were often associated with this procedure[43]. Subsequently, a more advanced technique attempting to isolate the PV muscle sleeves form the left atrium evolved.

Among various procedures to isolate the PV muscle sleeves from the LA initially employed by several investigators, two approaches predominated: namely, segmental ostial ablation at sites where localized conductions between the PV and the LA were electrophysiologically identified[44], and anatomically guided circumferential PV ablation encircling individual PVs[45].

Presently, almost all centers empirically isolate all four PVs not at the ostium but outside the tubular portion of the PV to avoid the risk of venous stenosis and improve procedural efficacy. Because the PV is funnel-shaped with a large proximal end (referred to as the antrum), which blends into the posterior wall of the LA, isolation of the PV and the surrounding antral tissue has become the current goal of this procedure.

In order to eliminate the substrate for maintaining AF, the efficiency of two additional adjunctive ablation strategies of PV isolation have been described. The linear lesions are made at the roof between the contralateral superior PVs (roof line) and at the isthmus between the mitral valve and the left inferior PV (mitral isthmus line) [46, 47]. This concept improved the AF-free ratio from 69 to 87% in paroxysmal AF cases, although epicardial RF applications were required in 60% of cases to achieve the mitral isthmus block.

Currently, the most popular method for AF substrate modification in the atrium is to apply RF energy and create lesions targeting the areas with complex fractionated atrial electrograms (CFAEs) [48]. CFAEs are believed to represent slow conduction or pivot points where wavelets turn around at the end of arcs of functional blocks. Although the concept of this method is well accepted, its role in ablation strategies has not yet been fully established. CFAE ablation targets only the substrate to perpetuate AF, and only modest efficacy of this method alone for chronic AF has been reported so far[49]. More recently, CFAE ablation has been achieving a general consensus as one of the combination strategies for modifying AF substrates.

Ablation treatment is successful in approximately 60% to 70% of patients that 10% to 40% of patients require a second ablation procedure, and that 10% to 15% still need antiarrhythmic drugs[50].

Success rates for catheter-based ablation are lower in patients with persistent atrial fibrillation than in those with paroxysmal AF. In addition, the chances of a successful outcome are lower in those with marked dilation of the left atrium. Oral and colleagues51 reported 75% recurrence rate in patients with persistent AF, compared with 29% in patients with paroxysmal AF.

4.8 Ablation strategy for chronic atrial fibrillation

Multiple strategies of various procedures, including PV isolation, anatomy- or electrogram-guided left-atrial ablation, linear ablation and thoracic vein isolation, have been developed. Each strategy performed alone has been shown to yield similar rates of outcome (50–70% success), suggesting the various co-existing targets and factors as the modifiers of the AF substrates. Haïssaguerre et al. developed stepwise multifaceted ablation method for chronic AF, which could integrate different (electrogram- and anatomy based) approaches[55-57]. They combined the approaches of PV isolation, electrogram-based ablation targeting CFAEs, linear ablation at the LAroof and the mitral isthmus and right atrial ablation (in some cases). Up to now, no single strategy is uniformly effective in patients with persistent and long-standing persistent AF.

4.9 Indication for catheter ablation

Catheter ablation should generally not be the first-line therapy for atrial fibrillation. The primary indication for it is symptomatic atrial fibrillation that is refractory to at least one class 1 or class 3 antiarrhythmic drug or the inability of a patient to tolerate these drugs. Another indication is in patients in whom rapid atrial fibrillation is determined to be the cause of tachycardia-mediated cardiomyopathy resulting in heart failure, reduced ejection fraction, or both. Studies have been performed in which catheter ablation was used as first-line therapy. The expert consensus committee[2] recognized this but did not fully support the practice. The decision to proceed with catheter ablation must be individualized on the basis of the risk of complications, the likely benefits, and the likelihood of success.

Recent guidelines have class I recommendation for ablation in selected patients with significantly symptomatic paroxysmal AF and failed treatment with an antiarrhythmic drug and have normal or mildly dilated left atria, normal or mildly reduced LV function, and no severe pulmonary disease, when performed in experienced centers.

An absolute contraindication to catheter ablation is left atrial thrombus. Because of the risk of dislodging an existing thrombus during the procedure and causing a stroke, patients with persistent atrial fibrillation who are in atrial fibrillation at the time of the procedure should undergo trans esophageal echocardiography to screen for thrombus.

4.10 Complications of RFA

The most common complication associated with catheter ablation of AF is symptomatic or asymptomatic pulmonary vein stenosis (defined as a >70% reduction in lumen diameter), with an overall incidence of 1.6%. Somewhat less common are cardiac tamponade (0.7%), pericardial effusion (0.6%), periprocedural stroke (0.3%), and periprocedural transient ischemic attack (0.2%). The overall mortality rate is 0.7%[58].

It is clear that catheter ablation is more effective than AAD therapy in treating AF. However because of associated complication catheter ablation of AF should be considered after a patient has failed attempts at treatment with 1 or more AAD.

4.11 The surgical maze procedure

Surgeons were the first ones to treat AF effectively and reverse it to sinus rhythm. James Cox described a series of surgical procedures known as Cox-Maze technique. The maze procedure is based on the concept that a critical mass of atrial tissue is needed to allow multiple waves of depolarisation to spread. This surgical approach was directed to divide both right and left atria by a series of cuts and sutures to redirect the electrical impulse to close-end paths. This operation also included the exclusion of both atrial appendages and the isolation of the four pulmonary veins and the posterior wall of the left atrium. Nowadays, cryotherapy, bipolar radiofrequency, and ultrasounds are the most used energy sources.

Although very effective, with over 91% patients maintaining sinus rhythm at 10 years, few surgical groups performed the Cox-Maze procedure due to the aggressiveness of it, with long suture lines and prolonged myocardial ischemic times[59,60]. Preoperative AF is associated with worse survival rates after valvular or coronary surgery. Furthermore, patients with successful maze procedures have shown better long-term survival rates, higher freedom from stroke, and thromboembolic events, improved ventricular ejection fraction and exercise tolerance. All the above factors have expanded the indications for the surgical treatment of concomitant AF to most patients with coronary or valvular surgery.

In addition, minimally invasive approaches have been described in the last five years with very good results for isolated paroxysmal or persistent AF. Nevertheless, prospective randomized trials are necessary to confirm their long-term results, compared to catheter ablation.

4.12 Pacing for atrial fibrillation

Atrial-based pacing, in either single- or dual-chamber mode, reduced the incidence of AF in several prospective multicenter studies[62-67]. More recently, a variety of preventive atrial pacing strategies, including continuous overdrive pacing, pacing in response to atrial premature beats, postmode switch and postexercise pacing therapies, were developed to reduce the burden of AF among patients with known atrial tachyarrhythmias[68-73].

However, the magnitude of AF prevention due to dedicated preventive pacing algorithms and the identification of responder candidates remains unclear[74-76].

4.13 Atrioventricular node ablation

Atrioventricular (AV) node ablation provides highly effective control of ventricular rate in patients with AF. Catheter ablation of AV node is a palliative but irreversible procedure and is therefore reasonable in patients in whom pharmacological rate control, or rhythm control with drugs and/or ablation therapy has failed. In such patients, AV node ablation improves quality of life and renders mortality similar to death rates in the general population. It is reasonable to assume that patients with LV systolic dysfunction may require biventricular pacing after AV node ablation to prevent deterioration of LV function. In patients without LV dysfunction, it is not established at present whether biventricular pacing is needed: some data suggest that biventricular pacing may be beneficial,[77] while others demonstrate similar benefits with right ventricular pacing.

4.14 Obliteration of the left atrial appendage

The left atrial appendage (LAA) is considered the main site of atrial thrombogenesis.Thus, occlusion of the LAA may therefore be an effective way to reduce thromboembolic risk. Surgical closure is recommended only as an adjunctive procedure in patients undergoing mitral valve surgery. However devices have been developed that allows percutaneous LAA closure via the transeptal approach. This may be appropriate for patients who are not suitable for anticoagulation[78]. Further trials are needed to evaluate its long term safety and efficacy.

4.15 Rheumatic valvular heart disease and atrial fibrillation

AF is frequently associated with rheumatic valvular heart disease (RVHD). Valvular heart disease is one of risk factors for development of AF. The frequency of RVHD has decreased in developed but RVHD constitutes a significant burden on healthcare in developing countries.

The risk of thromboembolism in patients with RVHD and AF is high. The stroke risk increases 17-fold if patients have rheumatic heart disease and AF, compared with age-matched controls[79]. AF worsens hemodynamics in patients with RVHD as absent atrial kick and irregular ventricular rhythm lead to a fall in cardiac output.

Results of randomized trials evaluating strategies for heart rate control or rhythm control is not necessarily acceptable for patients with RVHD and AF, because the majority of patients in these trials were non-RVHD. In patients with RVHD and AF, the maintenance of sinus rhythm can be expected to improve mortality and QOL. It is suggested that in RVHD and AF if there is no significant valvular compromise necessitating intervention and if the left atrium size is not more than 6.0 cms, rhythm control with amiodarone facilitated by electrical cardioversions should be the strategy[82]. If attempts to maintain SR fail over one year's time, rate control measures should suffice In young patients and those with RVHD but no significant valve compromise, restoring and maintaining SR should be attempted.

Patients receiving mechanical valve replacement need to continue anticoagulant therapy. It is unclear whether or not the maintenance of sinus rhythm influences clinical outcome for thromboembolism in these patients. However, the maintenance of sinus rhythm is important patients receiving tissue valve replacement, or balloon intervention, because they are likely to discontinue anticoagulant therapy.

If AF persists, electrical and pharmacologic cardioversion are effective in restoring sinus rhythm, and the administration of antiarrhythmic drugs may be effective in preventing

AF[80]. However, once AF has developed in patients with RVHD, these drugs may not be effective in restoring sinus rhythm because of the pathological changes that develop in the atrium and predispose to AF.

Surgery for AF should be utilized for patients with associated RVHD undergoing valve surgery. The probability of spontaneous conversion to SR after isolated mitral valve surgery is less than 10%. Patients who return to SR after mitral valve replacement or repair demonstrate better survival and freedom from adverse events.

After the success of the Cox maze III procedure in treating AF, several surgeons began to add the maze procedure as an adjunct to mitral valve surgery to treat both problems[81]. Successful restoration of SR has been achieved in 70-96% of patients.

5. Conclusion

Recent developments in pharmacological and non-pharmacological therapy have opened a new horizon in management of AF. Cure of AF has, however become a realistic goal albeit in limited number of patients and will remain a challenge for years to come.

6. References

[1] Wyse DG, Waldo AL, DiMarco JP, Domanski MJ, Rosenberg Y, Schron EB, Kellen JC, Greene HL, Mickel MC, Dalquist JE, Corley SD; Atrial fibrillation follow-up investigation of rhythm management (AFFIRM) investigators. A comparison of rate control and rhythm control in patients with atrial fibrillation. N Engl J Med 2002;347:1825-1833.

[2] Calkins H, Brugada J, Packer DL, et al. HRS/EHRA/ECAS expert consensus statement on catheter and surgical ablation of atrial fibrillation: recommendations for personnel, policy, procedures and follow-up. A report of the Heart Rhythm Society (HRS) Task Force on Catheter and Surgical Ablation of Atrial Fibrillation developed in partnership with the European Heart Rhythm Association (EHRA) and the European Cardiac Arrhythmia Society (ECAS); in collaboration with the American College of Cardiology (ACC), American Heart Association (AHA), and the Society of Thoracic Surgeons (STS). Endorsed and approved by the governing bodies of the American College of Cardiology, the American Heart Association, the European Cardiac Arrhythmia Society, the European Heart Rhythm Association, the Society of Thoracic Surgeons, and the Heart Rhythm Society. Europace 2007; 9:335–379.

[3] Haissaguerre M, Jais P, Shah DC, Takahashi A, Hocini M, Quiniou G, et al. Spontaneous initiation of atrial fibrillation by ectopic beats originating in the pulmonary veins. N Engl J Med 1998;339: 659–66.

[4] Tsai CF, Tai CT, Hsieh MH, Lin WS, Yu WC, Ueng KC, et al. Initiation of atrial fibrillation by ectopic beats originating from the superior vena cava: electrophysiological characteristics and results of radiofrequency ablation. Circulation 2000;102:67–74.

[5] Hwang C, Karagueuzian HS, Chen PS. Idiopathic paroxysmal atrial fibrillation induced by a focal atr discharge mechanism in the left superior pulmonary vein: possible roles of the ligament of Marshall. J Cardiovasc Electrophysiol 1999;10:636–48.

[6] Allessie MA, Konings K, Kirchhof CJ, Wijffels M. Electrophysiologic mechanisms of perpetuation of atrial fibrillation. Am J Cardiol 1996; 77: 10–23A.

[7] Fareh S, Villemaire C, Nattel S. Importance of refractoriness heterogeneity in the enhanced vulnerability to atrial fibrillation induction caused by tachycardia-induced atrial electrical remodeling. Circulation 1998;98:2202–9.
[8] Singh J, Braich JS. Recent advances in pharmacotherapy of atrial fibrillation. Indian J Pharmacol 2009;41:153-157.
[9] Bajpai A, Savelieva I, Camm AJ. Treatment of atrial fibrillation. Br Med Bull 2008;88:75-94
[10] Van Gelder IC, Crijns HJ, Tieleman RG, Brugemann J, De Kam PJ, Gosselink AT, et al. Chronic atrial fibrillation: success of serial cardioversion therapy and safety of oral anticoagulation. Arch Intern Med 1996; 156: 2585–92
[11] Volgman AS, Soble JS, Neumann A, Mukhtar KN, Iftikhar F, Vallesteros A, et al. Effect of left atrial size on recurrence of atrial fibrillation after electrical cardioversion: atrial dimension versus volume. Am J Card Imaging 1996;10:261–5.
[12] Consensus Conference on Atrial Fibrillation in Hospital and General Practice. Final consensus statement. Proc R Coll Physicians Edinb 1999;suppl 6: 2–3.
[13] Albers GW, Dalen JE, Laupacis A, Manning WJ, Petersen P, Singer DE. Antithrombotic therapy in atrial fibrillation. Stroke 2001; 119: 194–206S.
[14] Wyse DG, Waldo AL, DiMarco JP, Domanski MJ, Rosenberg Y, Schron EB, Kellen JC, Greene HL, Mickel MC, Dalquist JE, Corley SD; Atrial fibrillation follow-up investigation of rhythm management (AFFIRM) investigators. A comparison of rate control and rhythm control in patients with atrial fibrillation. N Engl J Med 2002;347:1825-1833.
[15] Martinez-Marcos FJ, Garcia-Garmendia JL, Ortega-Carpio A, Fernandez-Gomez JM, Santos JM, Camacho C. Comparison of intravenous flecainide, propafenone, and amiodarone for conversion of acute atrial fibrillation to sinus rhythm. Am J Cardiol 2000;86:950–3.
[16] Roy D, Pratt CM, Torp-Pedersen C, Wyse DG, Toft E, Juul-Moller S, et al. Vernakalant hydrochloride for rapid conversion of atrial fibrillation: a phase 3, randomized, placebo-controlled trial. Circulation. 2008 Mar 25;117(12):1518-25.
[17] Kowey PR, Dorian P, Mitchell LB, Pratt CM, Roy D, Schwartz PJ, et al. Vernakalant hydrochloride for the rapid conversion of atrial fibrillation after cardiac surgery: a randomized, double-blind, placebo-controlled trial. Circ Arrhythm Electrophysiol
[18] Alboni P, Botto GL, Baldi N, Luzi M, Russo V, Gianfranchi L, Marchi P,Calzolari M, Solano A, Baroffio R, Gaggioli G. Outpatient treatment of recent-onset atrial fibrillation with the 'pill-in-the-pocket' approach. N Engl J Med 2004;351:2384–2391.
[19] Van Gelder IC, Crijns HJ, Van Gilst WH, Verwer R, Lie KI. Prediction of uneventful cardioversion and maintenance of sinus rhythm from direct-current electrical cardioversion of chronic atrial fibrillation and flutter. Am J Cardiol 1991;68:41–6.
[20] Doyle JF, Ho KM. Benefits and risks of long-term amiodarone therapy for persistent atrial fibrillation: a meta-analysis. Mayo Clin Proc 2009;84:234-342.
[21] Le Heuzey JY, De Ferrari GM, Radzik D, et al. A Short-Term, Randomized,Double-Blind, Parallel-Group Study to Evaluate the Efficacy and Safety of Dronedarone versus Amiodarone in Patients with Persistent Atrial Fibrillation:The DIONYSOS Study. J Cardiovasc Electrophysiol. 2010;21:597- 605.
[22] Hohnloser SH, Crijns HJ, van Eickels M: for the ATHENA Investigators. Effectof dronedarone on cardiovascular events in atrial fibrillation N Engl J Med. 2009;360:668–78.

[23] Bernard EO, Schmid ER, Schmidlin D, Scharf C, Candinas R, Germann R. Ibutilide versus amiodarone in atrial fibrillation: a double-blinded, randomized study. Crit Care Med 2003;31:1031-1034.
[24] Giudici MC, Fischer WJ 3rd, Cervantes DC, Schrumpf PE, Paul DL, Sentman KE, Serra VL, Barold SS. Ibutilide therapy for atrial fibrillation: 5-Year experience in a community hospital. J Cardiovasc Nurs 2008;23:484-488.
[25] Torp-Pedersen C, Moller M, Kober L, Camm AJ. Dofetilide for the treatment of atrial fibrillation in patients with congestive heart failure. Eur Heart J 2000;21:1204-1206.
[26] Køber L, Torp-Pedersen C, McMurray JJ, Gøtzsche O, Lévy S, Crijns H, Amlie J, Carlsen J; Dronedarone study group. Increased mortality after dronedarone therapy for severe heart failure. N Engl J Med 2008;358:2678-2687.
[27] Fuster V, Rydén LE, Cannom DS, Crijns HJ, Curtis AB, Ellenbogen KA, Halperin JL, Heuzey JYL, Kay GN, Lowe JE, Olsson SB, Prystowsky EN, Tamargo JL, Wann S. ACC/AHA/ESC 2006 Guidelines for the Management of Patients with Atrial FibrillationExecutive Summary. JACC 2006;48:854-906.
[28] Segal OR. Rate control for atrial fibrillation: one drug or two? Postgrad 2009;85:281-282.
[29] Van Gelder IC, Groenveld HF, Crijns HJ, et al. Lenient versus strict rate control in patients with atrial fibrillation. N Engl J Med. 2010;362:1363–73.
[30] Freudenberger RS, Wilson AC, Kostis JB; AFFIRM investigators and committees. Comparison of rate versus rhythm control for atrial fibrillation in patients with left ventricular dysfunction (from the AFFIRM study). Am J Cardiol 2007;100:247-252.
[31] Van Gelder IC, Hagens VE, Bosker HA, Kingma JH, Kamp O, Kingma T, Said SA, Darmanata JI, Timmermans AJ, Tijssen JG, Crijns HJ; Rate control versus electrical cardioversion for persistent atrial fibrillation study group. A comparison of rate control and rhythm control in patients with recurrent persistent atrial fibrillation. N Engl J Med 2002;347:1834-1840.
[32] Hohnloser SH, Kuck KH, Lilienthal J. Rhythm or rate control in atrial fibrillation pharmacological intervention in atrial fibrillation (PIAF): a randomized trial. Lancet 2000;356:1789-1794.2
[33] Nieuwlaat R, Prins MH, Le Heuzey JY, Vardas PE, Aliot E, Santini M, Cobbe SM Widdershoven JW, Baur LH, Levy S, Crijns HJ. Prognosis, disease progression, and treatment of atrial fibrillation patients during 1 year: follow-up of the Euro heart survey on atrial fibrillation. Eur Heart J 2008;29:1181-1189
[34] Thambidorai SK, Murray RD, Parakh K, Shah TK, Black IW, Jasper SE, Li J, Apperson-Hansen C, Asher CR, Grimm RA, Klein AL; ACUTE investigators. Utility of transesophageal echocardiography in identification of thrombogenic milieu in patients with atrial fibrillation (an ACUTE ancillary study). Am J Cardiol 2005;96:935-941.
[35] Kavlak ES, Kucukoglu H, Yigit Z, Okcun B, Baran T, Ozkan AA, Kucukoglu S. Clinical and echocardiographic risk factors for embolization in the presence of left atrial thrombus. Echocardiography 2007;24:515-521.
[36] Fuster V, Ryden LE, Asinger RW, Cannom DS, Crijns HJ, Frye RL, et al. ACC/AHA/ESC guidelines for the management of patients with atrial fibrillation: a report of the American College of Cardiology/American Heart Association Task Force on Practice Guidelines and the European Society of Cardiology Committee for Practice Guidelines and Policy Conferences (committee to develop guidelines for the management of patients with atrial fibrillation) developed in collaboration

with the North American Society of Pacing and Electrophysiology. Eur Heart J 2001; 22: 1852–923

[37] Menke J, Lüthje L, Kastrup A, Larsen J. Thromboembolism in atrial fibrillation. Am J Cardiol 2010;105:502-510.

[38] Connolly S, Pogue J, Hart R, et al. Clopidogrel plus aspirin versus oral anticoagulation for atrial fibrillation in the Atrial fibrillation Clopidogrel Trial with Irbesartan for prevention of Vascular Events (ACTIVE W): a randomized controlled trial. Lancet. 2006;367:1903–12.

[39] Connolly SJ, Pogue J, Hart RG, et al. Effect of clopidogrel added to aspirin in patients with atrial fibrillation. N Engl J Med. 2009;360:2066 –78.

[40] Connolly SJ, Ezekowitz MD, Yusuf S, Eikelboom J, Oldgren J, Parekh A, Pogue J, Reilly PA, Themeles E, Varrone J, Wang S, Alings M, Xavier D, Zhu J, Diaz R, Lewis BS, Darius H, Diener HC, Joyner CD, Wallentin L; RE-LY steering committee and investigators. Dabigatran versus warfarin in patients with atrial fibrillation. N Engl J Med 2009;361:1139-1151.

[41] Connolly S J, Eikelboom J, Joyner C, Franzosi M G, et al, AVERROES Steering Committee and Investigators. N Engl J Med 2011 ; 364 : 806-817.

[42] Corley SD, Epstein AE, DiMarco JP, Domanski MJ, Geller N, Greene HL, Josephson RA, Kellen JC, Klein RC, Krahn AD, Mickel M, Mitchell LB, Nelson JD, Rosenberg Y, Schron E, Shemanski L, Waldo AL, Wyse DG: Relationships between sinus rhythm, treatment, and survival in the Atrial Fibrillation Follow-up Investigation of Rhythm Management (AFFIRM) study. Circulation 2004;109:1509-1513.

[43] Robbins IM, Colvin EV, Doyle TP, Kemp WE, Loyd JE, McMahon WS, Kay GN. Pulmonary vein stenosis after catheter ablation of atrial fibrillation. Circulation. 1998;98:1769–75.

[44] HaïssaguerreM, Shah DC, Jaïs P, et al. Electrophysiological breakthroughs from the left atrium to the pulmonary veins. Circulation. 2000;102:2463–2465

[45] Pappone C, Rosanio S, Oreto G, Tocchi M, Gugliotta F, Vicedomini G, Salvati A, et al. Circumferential radiofrequency ablation of pulmonary vein ostia: A new anatomic approach for curing atrial fibrillation. Circulation 2000;102:2619-2628.

[46] Hocini M, Jaïs P, Sanders P, Takahashi Y, Rotter M, Rostock T, et al. Techniques, evaluation, and consequences of linear block at the left atrial roof in paroxysmal atrial fibrillation: a prospective randomized study. Circulation. 2005;112:3688-96.

[47] Jais P, Hocini M, Hsu LF, et al. Technique and results of linear ablation at the mitral isthmus Circulation 2004;110:2996-3002.

[48] Nademanee K, McKenzie J, Kosar E, et al. A new approach for catheter ablation of atrial fibrillation: mapping of the electrophysiologic substrate. J Am Coll Cardiol 2004;43:2044 –53

[49] Oral H, Chugh A, Good E, Wimmer A, Dey S, Gadeela N, et al. Radiofrequency catheter ablation of chronic atrial fibrillation guided by complex electrograms. Circulation (2007) 115:2606-12.

[50] Crandall MA, Bradley DJ, Packer DL, Asirvatham SJ. Contemporary management of atrial fibrillation: update on anticoagulation and invasive management strategies. Mayo Clin Proc 2009; 84:643–662.

[51] Oral H, Knight BP, Tada H, et al. Pulmonary vein isolation for paroxysmal and persistent atrial fibrillation. Circulation 2002; 105:1077–1081.

[52] Wazni OM, Marrouche NF, Martin DO, et al. Radiofrequency ablation vs antiarrhythmic drugs as first-line treatment of symptomatic atrial fibrillation: a randomized trial. JAMA 2005; 293:2634–2640.
[53] Jaïs P, Cauchemez B, Macle L, et al. Catheter ablation versus antiarrhythmic drugs for atrial fibrillation: the A4 study. Circulation 2008; 118:2498–2505.
[54] Pappone C, Augello G, Sala S, et al. A randomized trial of circumferential pulmonary vein ablation versus antiarrhythmic drug therapy in paroxysmal atrial fibrillation: the APAF Study. J Am Coll Cardiol 2006; 48:2340–2347.
[55] Haïssaguerre M, Sanders P, Hocini M, et al., J Cardiovasc Electrophysiol, 2005;16:1125–37.
[56] Jaïs P, O'Neill MD, Takahashi Y, et al., J Cardiovasc Electrophysiol, 2006;17(Suppl. 3):S28–36.
[57] Matsuo S, Lim KT, Haïssaguerre M, Heart Rhythm,2007;4:1461–3.
[58] Calkins H, Reynolds MR, Spector P, et al. Treatment of atrial fibrillation with antiarrhythmic drugs or radiofrequency ablation: two systematic literature reviews and meta-analyses. Circ Arrhythm Electrophysiol. 2009;2:349–61
[59] J. L. Cox, "The surgical treatment of atrial fibrillation: IV.Surgical technique," Journal of Thoracic and Cardiovascular Surgery, vol. 101, no. 4, pp. 584–592, 1991.
[60] J. L. Cox, J. P. Boineau, R. B. Schuessler, R. D. Jaquiss, and D. G. Lappas, "Modification of the maze procedure for atrial flutter and atrial fibrillation. I. Rationale and surgical results,Journal of Thoracic and Cardiovascular Surgery, vol. 110, no. 2,pp. 473–484, 1995.
[61] E. Lim, C. W. Barlow, A. R. Hosseinpour et al., "Influence of atrial fibrillation on outcome following mitral valve repair,"
[62] Lamas GA, Lee KL, Sweeney MO, et al, for the Mode Selection Trial in Sinus Node Dysfunction Investigators. Ventricular pacing or dual-chamber pacing for sinus-node dysfunction. N Engl J Med 2002;346:1854 –1862.
[63] Kerr CR, Connolly SJ, Abdollah H, et al, for the Canadian Trial of Physiological Pacing (CTOPP) Investigators. Canadian Trial of Physiologic Pacing: effects of physiologic pacing during long-term follow-up. Circulation 2004;109:357–362.
[64] Connolly SJ, Kerr CR, Gent M, et al. Effects of physiologic pacing versus ventricular pacing on the risk of stroke and death due to cardiovascular causes. Canadian Trial of Physiologic Pacing Investigators. N Engl J Med 2000;342:1385–1391.
[65] Andersen HR, Nielsen JC, Thomsen PE, et al. Long-term follow-up of patients from a randomized trial of atrial versus ventricular pacing for sick sinus syndrome. Lancet 1997;350:1210 –1216.
[66] Delfaut P, Saksena S, Prakash A, et al. Long-term outcome of patients with drug-refractory atrial flutter and fibrillation after single-and dual-site right atrial pacing for arrhythmia prevention. J Am Coll Cardiol 1998;32:1900 –1908.
[67] Lamas GA, Orav EJ, Stambler BS, et al. Quality of life and clinical outcomes in elderly patients treated with ventricular pacing as compared with dual-chamber pacing. Pacemaker Selection in the Elderly Investigators. N Engl J Med 1998;338:1097–104.
[68] Blanc JJ, De Roy L, Mansourati J, et al, for the PIPAF Investigators. Atrial pacing for prevention of atrial fibrillation: assessment of simultaneously implemented algorithms. Europace 2004;6:371–379.
[69] Lee MA, Weachter R, Pollak S, et al. The effect of atrial pacing therapies on atrial tachyarrhythmia burden and frequency: results of a randomized trial in patients with bradycardia and atrial tachyarrhythmias. J Am Coll Cardiol 2003;41:1926 –1932.

[70] Padeletti L, Purerfellner H, Adler SW, et al, for the Worldwide ASPECT Investigators. Combined efficacy of atrial septal lead placement and atrial pacing algorithms for prevention of paroxysmal atrial tachyarrhythmia. J Cardiovasc Electrophysiol 2003;14:1189 -1195.

[71] Levy T, Walker S, Rex S, et al. Does atrial overdrive pacing prevent paroxysmal atrial fibrillation in paced patients? Int J Cardiol 2000;75:91–97.

[72] Lozano IF, Vincent A, Roda J, et al. Paroxysmal atrial fibrillation prevention by pacing in patients with pacemaker indication. Europace 2003;5:267–273.

[73] Israel CW, Hohnloser SH. Pacing to prevent atrial fibrillation. J Cardiovasc Electrophysiol 2003;14(9 Suppl):S20 -S26.

[74] Carlson MD, Ip J, Messenger J, et al. A new pacemaker algorithm for the treatment of atrial fibrillation: results of the Atrial Dynamic Overdrive Pacing Trial (ADOPT). J Am Coll Cardiol 2003;42:627- 633.

[75] Knight BP, Gersh BJ, Carlson MD, et al, for the AHA Writing Group. Role of permanent pacing to prevent atrial fibrillation: science advisory from the AHA Council on Clinical Cardiology and the Quality of Care and Outcomes Research Interdisciplinary Working Group, in collaboration with the Heart Rhythm Society. Circulation 2005;111:240 -243.

[76] Savelieva I, Camm AJ. The results of pacing trials for the prevention and termination of atrial tachyarrhythmias: is there any evidence of therapeutic breakthrough? J Interv Card Electrophysiol 2003;8:103–115.

[77] Gasparini M, Auricchio A, Metra M, Regoli F, Fantoni C, Lamp B, Curnis A,Vogt J, Klersy C. Long-term survival in patients undergoing cardiac resynchronization therapy: the importance of performing atrio-ventricular junction ablation in patients with permanent atrial fibrillation. Eur Heart J 2008;29:1644–1652.

[78] Holmes DR, Reddy VY, Turi ZG, Doshi SK, Sievert H, Buchbinder M, Mullin CM,Sick P. Percutaneous closure of the left atrial appendage versus warfarin therapy for prevention of stroke in patients with atrial fibrillation: a randomised noninferiority trial. Lancet 2009;374:534–542.

[79] Wolf P, Dawber T, Thomas HJ, et al. Epidemiologic assessment of chronic atrial fibrillation and risk of stroke: the Framingham study. Neurology. 1978;28(10):973-977.

[80] Vora A, Karnad D, Goyal V, Naik A, Gupta A, Lokhandwala Y, et al. Control of rate versus rhythm in rheumatic atrial fibrillation: a randomized study. Indian Heart J 2004; 56: 110-116.

[81] Khargi K, Hutten BA, Lemke B, Deneke T. Surgical treatment of atrial fibrillation: a systemic review. Eur J Cardiothorac Surg 2005; 27: 258-265.

[82] Vora A. Management of atrial fibrillation in rheumatic valvular heart disease. Curr Opin Cardiol 2006; 21: 47-50.

7

Trends in Degenerative Aortic Disease: Novel Alternative Therapies for the Treatment of Severe Aortic Stenosis

Javier Gualis, Alejandro Diego, Antonio de Miguel and Mario Castaño
Complejo Hospitalario Universitario de León, Spain

1. Introduction

Aortic stenosis is the most common valvular disease among the occidental population and it is one of the most important causes of morbidity and mortality in developed countries. It has an incidence of 4% among over 80 years old patients (Charlson E et al.,2006). Its evolution is generally slowly progressive from asymptomatic/mild aortic stenosis to the symptomatic/severe form when survival is dramatically reduced as well as quality of live is importantly impaired. (Iung B et al., 2003)

All along natural history of this disease, patients will consult several times to specialists in order to adjust medical treatment and perform the indicated diagnostic tests. Occasionally in-hospital admittance will be unavoidable and this will necessarily arise into economic resources consumption, that might be assumed by actually over-the-edge and almost bankrupted socio-sanitary policies, at least in the most of developed countries (Varadarajan P, 2006; Pai RG, 2006).

Over more tan 40 years, standard treatment for severe symptomatic aortic stenosis has been focused in surgical replacement of the affected valve for a mechanical prosthesis. To achieve this replacement, patient must mandatorily undergo several risky procedures as general anesthesia, median sternotomy, and aortic arch clamping and cardioplegic solution infusion in order to maintain cardiac arrest in diastole during the intervention, with the indispensable cardiopulmonary bypass pumping. (Kvidal P et al,. 2000)

Hence, standard surgical therapy has inherent morbi-mortality risks itself that must be carefully evaluated, so this therapy may be not suitable for a subpopulation of candidates because of an excessive high-risk profile. These patients must then admit the natural history of this disease with a terribly poor mid-term prognosis and elevated economic expenses for the system. (Alexander KP et al., 2000)

Socio-sanitary policies need to organize the diagnostic and therapeutic procedures in this cohort of patients in order to obtain the necessary balance that allow an adequate treatment with risk minimization achieving the best possible results with the lowest expenses, optimizing the efficiency in the management of these complex pathology.

In this moment, several therapeutic alternatives are being studied with the aim of the risk reduction in the management of patients with severe aortic stenosis and surgical high-risk profile. These therapies do not pretend to become a substitution of the standard surgical

therapy but a way to reduce the burden of complication and morbidity in the subgroup of patients that cannot be eligible for standard surgery. (Rodés-Cabau et al., 2008)
The present chapter is dedicated to a detailed description of the different therapeutic procedures that are being developed nowadays as an alternative to standard surgical treatment. Special surgical new techniques as low-profile mechanical prosthesis, biological prosthesis (both stented and stentless), homograft and Ross technique (pulmonary autograft in aortic position and homograft in pulmonary position) will not be commented in this chapter.

2. Aortic valvuloplasty

Aortic balloon valvuloplasty is a classical procedure firstly performed in the late fifties and still in use for children affected of congenital aortic stenosis with acceptable results. Its use in degenerative or rheumatic aortic stenosis has been abandoned in the last decades due to its prohibitive mid-term restenosis rates. With good results limited to the first days after procedure, generally approved indications for severe aortic stenosis has been displaced towards a bridging therapy between a critical clinical situation and a surgical replacement that is delayed for any cause. Other previous indications, as palliative therapy among patients that reject surgery, previous to non-cardiac surgery or low gradient aortic stenosis with severely reduced left ventricle ejection fraction are losing their sense with the introduction of transcatheter aortic valve implantation, but all the way this novel therapy requires aortic valve balloon dilatation previously to device implantation, balloon valvuloplasty is not only out of danger of disappear but be clearly reinforced, redirected towards its implication in the TAVI procedure process. (Vahanian A et al., 2004).

3. Transcatheter aortic valve implantation: TAVI

Andersen performed first experimental studies of transcatheter aortic valve implantation in the early nineties (Andersen et al., 1992). Afterwards, in year 2000, Bonhoeffer did the first in-human implantation of a percutaneous prosthesis in pulmonary position (Bonhoeffer P et al., 2000) , but it was not until 2002 when Dr. Alain Cribier performed successfully the first implantation in a patient affected of severe symptomatic aortic stenosis rejected for surgery, obtaining an excellent initial clinical result that led to a fast spreading of the technique and implementation of the devices (Cribier A ,. 2002). From this moment on, the development of valvular programs to perform catheter-based aortic stenosis treatment have been increasing exponentially worldwide.
In a summarized way, the procedure consists of the implantation of a biological prosthesis anchored in a metallic stent over the diseased and stenotic native valve using a percutaneous arterial and/or venous access or a transapical access after performing a minithoracotomy. All of these ways to access the aortic valve have the intention to avoid the median sternotomy and the cardiopulmonary bypass with its implicit risks.
First procedures were performed via catheterization of the femoral vein and accessing the right heart and then the aortic valve in an anterograde way through a transseptal puncture. Although this kind of procedure is still performed in selected patients, now the most frequently used technique is the retrograde method through arterial access described by Webb in 2005, using preferably femoral site of puncture, though subclavian or even ascending aorta itself can be performed to reach the aortic valve (Webb JG et al., 2006). The

transapical technique, described by Lichtenstein in 2006, would require surgical access with a minithoractomy and at this moment it is the second preferred method (Lichtenstein SV et al., 2006).

TAVI is a complex technique essentially reserved for very high perisurgical risk patients. It is important to emphasize that, due to its complexity, the learning curve of the technique must be performed following a strict program that minimize the risk of complications. Several groups have compared initial results with those obtained after the first learning curve period. Webb et al reported their experience after the first 168 Edwards Sapien transcatheter aortic valve implantation, both transfemoral (n=113) and transapical (n=55) showing a decrease in 30-days mortality from 14,3% in the first 84 patients to 8,3% in the second half of the sample. Of course, not only the experience acquirement but the technical advances in the device design have contributed to this results improvement (Webb JG et al., 2007). In the same line, Grube el al demonstrated a 73% reduction in 30-days mortality (from 40% to 10,8%) in 102 patients who underwent 18F CoreValve system valve implantation in comparison with an older sample treated with the first generation 25F device (Grube E et al ., 2005). This data suggest that, while improvements in the design of the device and the selection of patients keep on growing exponentially, a reduction in the learning curve requirements should be expected for the next generation of devices and future centre incorporations to this alternative technique.

Despite this technical improvements, they will never replace the importance of the learning curve. Himbert et al reported that, in relation with the initial experience of a specific centre, precisely the learning curve is the most important factor related to in-hospital mortality and mid-term survival after this kind of procedures. (Himbert D et al., 2009).

The most important issue for the generalization of these techniques is the indispensable device development carried out by the medical industry. The experimental tests performed by the different research and development programs have the goal of optimizing results by minimizing complications in the access site, increasing durability, improving flexibility and navigability of devices, developing non-traumatic guide-wires and catheters and low-profile stents that allow the active fixation of the valve and its homogeneous expansion in order to avoid paravalvular leaks and, at the end, improve general clinical results in terms of morbidity and mortality.

There are several devices commercialized, the most used are the Medtronic CoreValve® Transcatheter Aortic Valve Implantation System (Medtronic Inc, Minneapolis, USA) and the Edwards Sapien® Trancatheter Heart Valve system (Edwards Lifesciences Inc., Irvine, USA).

CoreValve first implantation was reported for Grube et al in 2005 and obtained the CE mark in 2007. More than 10.000 devices have been already successfully implanted in more than 34 countries, and recently a clinical trial has been approved by the Food and Drugs Administration to evaluate its results in the USA. At this time, this device is designed for a transarterial retrograde approach implantation. This device is made up of a porcine pericardium valve fixed to an auto-expandable nitinol stent designed to anchor both the outflow tract of the left ventricle and the ascending aorta. It is commercialized in two sizes: 26mm (indicated for aortic annulus between 20 and 23mm) and 29mm (for annulus between 23 and 27mm). It is delivered through a 18F sheath so it is intended to be used in patients with femoral artery diameters over 6mm.

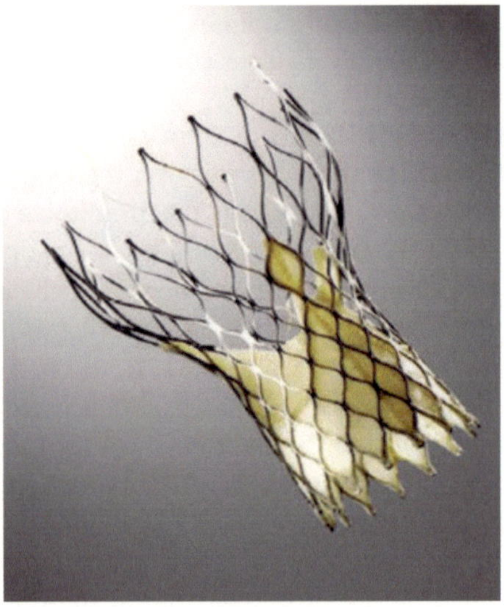

The Core Valve

The new Edwards Lifescience device, the Sapien-XT valve, can be delivered by an arterial or venous access site (anterograde or retrograde technique) as well as by a transapical approach; it has the CE mark since 2007 and has the FDA investigational device exemption for the PARTNER US trial. Like the CoreValve system, more than 10.000 devices have been implanted all around the world with promising initial results. It is constructed with a bovine pericardium valve sewed to a balloon expandable chromium-cobalt stent to be anchored to the calcified native aortic annulus. Three sizes are commercialized: 23mm (for aortic annulus between 18 and 21mm), 26mm (for aortic annulus between 21 and 25mm) and the recently added 29mm size for annulus over 25mm. The femoral sheath is 18F for the smaller size and 19F for the 26, and the transapical sheath is 22F for the smaller, 24F for the 26mm size and 26F for the 29mm. No femoral system has been designed yet for the 29mm valve.

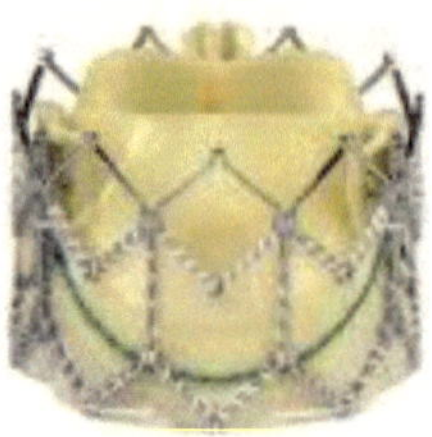

The Edwards Sapien XT valve

3.1 Indications

Initially, these devices were only approved as compassionate therapy for non operable patients with severe symptoms (NYHA class IV dyspnea or angina), but after the initial results achieved, the indications of these proceedings are extending to any patient with symptomatic severe aortic stenosis and specific contraindication for cardiac surgery or very high perioperative risk profile. It is reasonable to think that, as the technique is consolidating, the screening of patients for TAVI should follow the general recommendations for the management of patients with degenerative aortic stenosis reported by the scientific societies. (Vahanian A et al., 2007,2008)

3.1.1 General indications of aortic valve replacement for aortic stenosis following the European Society of Cardiology clinical guidelines

1. Patients with severe aortic stenosis and presence of any symptoms (Recommendation class IB).
2. Asymptomatic patients with severe aortic stenosis and systolic dysfunction (LVEF <50%) not attributable to other cause (IC).
3. Asymptomatic patients with severe aortic stenosis and exercise test that shows lowering of arterial systolic pressure under basal levels (IIaC).
4. Asymptomatic patients with severe aortic stenosis and severe calcification of the valve and a progression of the aortic peak velocity >0,3m/s per year (IIaC).
5. Patients with low gradient severe aortic stenosis (<40mmHg) with systolic dysfunction (LVEF<40%) and contractile reserve (IIaC).
6. Asymptomatic patients with severe aortic stenosis and exercise test that shows complex ventricular arrhythmias (IIbC).
7. Asymptomatic patients with severe aortic stenosis and left ventricle hypertrophy (>15mm) in case of no arterial hypertension (IIbC).
8. Patients with low gradient (<40mmHg) severe aortic stenosis and systolic dysfunction with no contractile reserve (IIbC).

   *Severe aortic stenosis is defined as a valvular area <1cm2 (<0,6cm2/m2 of body surface area) or a mean gradient >50mmHg with normal flow situation. Special evaluation is required in case of low flow situations.

3.1.2 Contraindication for conventional aortic valve replacement

1. High co-morbidity: elderly patients, left ventricle dysfunction, pulmonary hypertension, chronic obstructive pulmonary disease, renal failure, cerebrovascular disease, peripheral artery disease or any other circumstances evaluated following EuroSCORE (European System for Cardiac Operative Risk Evaluation) or STS (Society of Thoracic Surgeons) scales that leads to very high-risk profiles.
2. Excessive technical complexity: multiple re-interventions or porcelain aorta.

3.1.3 Absence of specific contraindications for transcatheter aortic valve implantation

In case of aortic valve replacement indication with contraindication for standard surgery or very high-risk patient, TAVI should be considered. If TAVI is indicated, because of slightly better mid-term clinical results (CITA), transarterial retrograde technique would be the preferred technique over the transapical approach, but always after taking into account the experience and/or preferences of the center.

- *General contraindications:*

1. Aortic annulus smaller than 18mm or bigger than 27mm.
2. Bicuspid or unicuspid aortic valve.
3. Asymmetric severe valve calcification (*bulky* calcification) that might lead to high risk of coronary ostia occlusion during implantation.
4. Severe symptomatic coronary artery disease not suitable for percutaneous revascularization.

5. Active infective endocarditis.
6. Hypertrophic Obstructive Myocardiopathy.

- *Contraindications for transfemoral access:*

1. Excessive tortuosity of the ilio-femoral axis.
2. Previous aorto-bifemoral by-pass surgery.
3. Small iliac or femoral artery diameter (<6-8mm depending on the device).
4. Severe angulation of proximal ascending aorta or the valvular plane.
5. Severe atheromatosis of ascending aorta or aortic arch, aortic coarctation, aneurism or dissection of descending thoracic aorta or abdominal aorta, specially if wall thrombus is present.
   *In case of TAVI indication and contraindication of femoral access, subclavian access might be considered.
   **In case of femoral/subclavian access contraindication, transapical access might be considered.

- *Contraindications for transapical access:*

1. Previous cardiac surgery on left ventricle apex.
2. Paricardium calcifications.
3. Chronic respiratory insufficiency that contraindicates minithoracotomy.
4. Apical thrombus in left ventricle.

3.2 TAVI program development

Before starting a new transcatheter program is essential to proceed with the organization of a local heart team that must be formed by two cardiothoracic surgeons, two interventional cardiologists, an echocardiographist, an anesthesiologist, two dedicated nurses, and a perfusionist. Problem-solving skills and learning ability are essential, as it is the collaboration among the different departments and units involved in order to front the complications that will arise during the learning curve.

Because of the elevated costs of the device, the difficulty of the technique and the high-risk profile of the candidates, specific learning courses realization is mandatory, as well as continuing training all along the team assistance trajectory. Industry demands, for both CoreValve and Sapien devices, a 15 procedures period in which the presence of a proctor that leads and trains the heart team is recommended before the achieving of the accreditation as an independent unit.

Patient screening must be performed with exquisite care as the success or failure of the starting program could depend on the results of the initial cases. We must never forget that elective therapy for severe aortic stenosis is still surgical replacement, and only when surgery is contraindicated or very risky TAVI can be considered. TAVI indication must be established after consensus between the heart team dedicated to this technique and the clinical cardiologist responsible of the candidate and not only clinical but economic criteria must be taken into account as the elevated expenses that this procedures involve requires the proper selection that may lead to optimal clinical long term results, both in terms of survival expectancy and quality of live.

Bullesfeld et al reported that pre-procedure patient functional class, assessed by Karnofsky index, was the only in-hospital survival predictor after CoreValve implantation. This fact comes to point again the main importance that an exhaustive screening process has in terms of late clinical results, and so in terms of efficiency (Bullesfeld L et al., 2009).

3.3 Additional diagnostic tests

Usual imaging complementary tests performed before TAVI are transthoracic echocardiography, transesophageal echocardiography, cardiac catheterization and coronary angiography and CT-scan and/or C-MRI. In addition to confirmation of aortic stenosis severity, detailed basic information is required regarding (Delgado V et al., 2010):

- Valve morphology (tricuspid or bicuspid, extend of calcification).
- Annulus diameter.
- Left ventricular outflow tract (LVOT) morphology.
- Morphology of the aortic root (sinuses and their relation to extensive valve calcification)
- Distance between coronary arteries and annulus (relation to sinus morphology and extensive valve calcification).
- Size, pathology (complex plaques, aneurysm) and course (kinking) of the entire aorta.
- Size, pathology (calcification) and course (tortuosity) of iliac and femoral arteries.

The consolidation of transcatheter aortic valve implantation procedures in the common practice will be related to the results obtained. Imaging techniques improvements and its application during the procedure can help to obtain better results. 3D-Transesophageal echocardiography will contribute with valuable information about device positioning, valve function and relation between the prosthesis and the coronary ostia and the aortic root. It is especially valuable in the assessment of leaflets calcifications that might cause early in-procedure complications during the valve deployment and will help the operator to find the proper positioning at the same time that allows identifying perivalvular leaks and guiding corrective manoeuvres in order to gain final prosthetic normal function and optimal performance. (Ng AC et al., 2010)

DynaCT is being introduced in the most advanced hybrid catheterization laboratories, adding a new tool that offers incomparable information about aortic root configuration and relations among the different structures involved in TAVI procedures, but at this moment, it is only available in a very few centres and, however in the next future it may become the usual guiding diagnostic tool, it cannot be considered as a standard requirement at this moment. (Kempfert J et al,. 2009)

3.4 Operating room

The ideal place to perform these complex techniques is called hybrid operating room or hybrid catheterization laboratory, were both, optimal x-ray imaging facilities and surgical treatment of the room adequate for cardiopulmonary by-pass, join together in order to minimize the risk of complications and adopt the necessary therapeutic measures in case of their presentation. The elevated cost of these hybrid rooms and the considerably big space that require make them to be out of reach for many centers, so several portable x-ray devices are being approved for its use into standard operating rooms.

3.5 Complications

Most often complication that may present in the early post-procedure period are: valve malposition, peri-prosthesis leak, acute aortic regurgitation and acute lung oedema, device embolization, low cardiac output heart failure with hemodynamic support requirements, conventional surgery conversion with in-pump connection, vascular access complications including vessel rupture, dissection and/or acute occlusion, stroke, myocardial infarction, coronary ostia occlusion, atrioventricular block and renal failure.

Valve malposition and valve embolization:

Valve malposition and valve embolization are classical complications very related to the different teams learning curve and the technical improvements in the deployment devices. They have been drastically reduced from initial series (approximately 6%) to the incidence reported in the pate trials (approximately 2%). (Walther T et al,. 2007)

Peri-prosthesis leak:

Peri-prosthesis leak is due to absence of complete apposition of the device to the aortic annulus caused by lack of homogeneous expansion and it is one of the most common complications and the most important factor related to post-procedural aortic regurgitation. This valve regurgitation, when it is severe, can generate acute hemodynamic instability and acute lung oedema (that also may appear after pre-implantation balloon valvuloplasty) and it is one of the most important issues to improve in order to achieve a real advance in this technique (Cribier A et al., 2006).

Vascular access complications:

Vascular access major complications are still over 10% in the majority of the series reported despite the results improvements. Experience with the CoreValve system indicates that transporter catheter diameter reduction has great impact in the reduction of these complications (from over 20% to 5% in the last registries). In addition to this, 22F catheter maintenance for Edwards Sapient system lead to a stabilization in the incidence of vascular complication despite the operators experience gaining. Anyway, it seems that, at least in the SOURCE registry, vascular complications do not determine higher 30-days mortality incidence. This suggests that the presence of highly prepared teams with experience in the treatment of these vascular complications may limit their impact in peri-procedural mortality.

It is important to advice that not only transfemoral technique is related to access complications as transapical access has also been associated with serious access complications as ventricular tear or severe bleeding during apex reparation. (Dumont E et al,. 2009, Rodés-Cabau J et al,. 2010)

Stroke:

Stroke, because of its terrible consequences for the patient, it has been another major concern of this technique. Stroke incidence has been kept below 5% in the majority of series; that is quite inferior to the expected incidence in an octogenarian population who undergo standard cardiac surgery with aortic clamping. This supports the idea that conventional aortic replacement surgery with cardiopulmonary by-pass and aortic clamping has a higher risk of stroke than these newer techniques despite the necessity of big sized aggressive devices that must navigate the aortic arch during implantation. It is important to remark here that transapical access avoids the manipulation of these catheters in the aorta and last trials have reported a tendency towards a stroke incidence reduction, so many centres have given priority to this access when severe aortic atheromatosis or porcelain aorta are present (Grube E et al,. 2008; Rodés-Cabau J et al,. 2010).

Myocardial infarction:

Assessing the incidence of myocardial infarction as a complication of TAVI is a very difficult objective as myocardial infarction definitions are quite variable among different trials and registries. Incidence vary from 0,2 to 17,5% depending on the definition given. In terms of severity and device-related myocardial infarction, the most important pathophysiological condition that must be watched is the occlusion of a coronary ostium secondary to calcified native valve leaflets displacement, much more frequent than ostium jailing phenomenon caused by the stent struts. Several groups have remark the importance of adequate assessment of the distance between the aortic annulus and coronary ostia to avoid this dramatic complication, especially in cases with severe calcifies native valve. Predicting peri-procedural myocardial infarction secondary to previous coronary disease would be much more difficult. Actually approved devices producers recommend the prophylaxis of this complication by coronary angiography and eventually percutaneous coronary intervention that should be performed at least 48 hours before TAVI. (Kapadia Sr et al,. 2009; Bagur R,. 2010; Wood D et al,. 2009)

Atriventricular block:

Atrioventricular block and need for pacemaker implantation has shown to be related to a low positioning of the valve that leads to His bundle conduction system injury. Incidence of permanent pacemaker implantation requirements after trancatheter valve implantation may vary among registries, but it looks clear that is much more frequent after CoreValve implantation in comparison with the Sapien system (10-33% vs <7%. (Piazza N et al,. 2008; Grube E et al., 2008). This difference is explained by the design characteristics of the CoreValve: the bigger length of the prosthesis favours under-aortic annulus anchorage and the nitinol autoexpandable alloy determines an additive progressive expansion of the stent after the deployment, with the subsequent risk of electric conduction system injury.

With such a high-risk of AV block, emphasis in the search for predictors that can anticipate the need for permanent pacemaker has been done. Jilahihawi et al recently reported the presence of previous left-bundle atrioventricular block, a ventricular septum bigger than 17mm or a non-coronary leaflet bigger than 8mm as a predictor for pacemaker requirement with a 75% sensibility and 100% specificity. (Jilahihawi H et al., 2009) Nevertheless, more studies with bigger sample sizes are needed before making definitive recommendations about prophylactic measures focused on avoiding this important, although rarely lethal, complication.

Advances in the knowledge of the aetiology and pathophysiologic generation of the atrioventricular block with different transcatheter valves will help to optimize final results. Alternative septum membranous anchorage systems that facilitate implantation on the native annulus and reduction of the terminal outflow tract cross-section size should be the key for improving results.

Renal failure and haemodialysis requirements:

Aregger et al evaluated the incidence of renal failure in a 54 patients cohort of CoreValve or Sapien implantation (Aregger F et al., 2009). The majority of the patients achieved an improvement in the creatinine serum levels after the procedure, but renal failure reached a 28% and 7,4% required haemodialysis during hospitalization. Bagur et al have recently reported a renal failure incidence of 11,7% after the Edwards Sapien device implantation, with a 4-fold in-hospital mortality increase (Bagur R et al., 2010). Curiously, in the same paper, incidence of acute renal failure among patients with previous chronic renal failure was lower in the group of TAVI than in the group of standard surgical valve replacement (9,2 vs 25,9%; haemodialysis requirements: 2,5 vs 8,7%).

3.6 Evidence

Degenerative aortic stenosis is a pathological process with stable prognosis and well known history for years, it can be considered as a "classical" heart disease and it has experimented very few advances during the past decades. Surgical valve replacement has shown itself as an excellent therapy and no alternative has arisen until the development of transcatheter valve implantation, and it has started its journey as a marginal palliative alternative for non-operable patients, so virtually no field for multicentre randomized double-blinded clinical trial that provide statistically reliable information that can guide evidence-based recommendations. Hence, the beginnings of transcatheter aortic valve implantation could be described at least as "complicated" and many difficulties have been overcome before achieving the minimal necessary strength before reaching the clinical trials era that now we are observing.

After initial heroic implantations performed by Cribier, Grub, Bonhoeffer or Webb, first experience was evaluated in several observational multicentre studies like SOURCE, REVIVE, REVIVE II and REVIVAL (Kodali SK et al., 2011). This studies reported valuable information about feasibility and safety of the technique with promising clinical results, but clinical randomized trials are needed before extracting definite conclusions about the true clinical benefits of transcatheter aortic valve implantation.

The SOURCE trial was a post-commercialization study in with the participation of 34 european centres that included a total of 463 patients with severe symptomatic aortic stenosis who underwent transfemoral aortic valve implantation because of severe comorbidities that made standard surgical therapy contraindicated or too risky. Immediate success of the procedure was achieved in 95,6% and 30-days after procedure survival was 93,7% in the whole cohort and 88,6% among patients who suffered vascular access complications. Other common complications reported were: pacemaker implantation (6,7%), aortic regurgitation > grade 2 (3,2%), device malaposition (1,7%) and coronary occlusion (0,7%). There was no device embolization event.(Wendler O et al., 2010; Thomas M et al., 2010)

After the initial results achieved during the first era and the spreading of the technique, major adverse cardiovascular events, in-hospital admittances, post-procedural functional class, complications, costs and quality of live are issues that must be contrasted no only against medical conservative therapy but also against conventional surgical treatment in this subset of high risk patients (but still considered operable). If clinical results still remain positive, long term follow-up and durability might be considered in order to extend clinical indication to lower risk profile patients.

After these first promising results it seems to be reasonable to affirm that TAVI is a feasible alternative to standard surgery for very high-risk patients, that allows offering them better expectative of survival and quality of life than a conservative pharmacological strategy.

In general, multicenter registries have included more than 2000 patients with an overall success over 90% and a 30-days mortality <10%, a definite step in order to confirm the feasibility, safety and efficacy of this technique as an alternative to surgical standard replacement in the subgroup of high-risk or prohibitive risk patients. At this point, direct comparison with surgical replacement does not look like a non-reachable objective, at least for the subgroup of patients in the frontier of the cardiopulmonary by-pass surgery indication (risk high enough to consider alternatives but not so much to be firmly rejected). This issue is the aim of the next generation of clinical trials involving TAVI.

In this way, the PARTNER trial pretends to give the response to these questions that initial practice arose. During the first part of this trial, patients with a diagnose of severe symptomatic aortic stenosis and rejected for surgery were randomly assigned into two groups: standard pharmacological conservative therapy or transcatheter aortic valve implantation. The results of this first step were reported in October 2010 and they showed a one-year mortality of 30,7% in the TAVI group vs 50,7% in the conservative therapy arm. Differences in hospital admission needs were as well statistically significant (42,5% in the TAVI group vs 71,6% in the conservative group) and a benefit in terms of functional class was observed too (NYHA class III/IV of 25,2% in TAVI group vs 58% in the pharmacological group), however, the incidence of stroke showed to be higher in the TAVI group (5% vs 1,1%) so they did vascular complications. (León MB et al., 2010)

Second part of PARTNER trial is actually on course and will try to compare the results of severe symptomatic aortic stenosis patients with very-high risk surgical profile randomly assigned into a group of standard surgical valve replacement or TAVI. Clinical events are being collected and publications of the results are expected for this year. They probably will guide the final clinical recommendations in the management of this complicated subgroup of patients.

Many individual and multicentre trials are on course at this moment trying to evaluate the efficiency of TAVI. As it is a novel technique in continuous evolution, European societies have recently published the guidelines to define the main endpoints that must be recorded in order to perform a conceptual standardization, that may serve as a reference for future comparisons among different studies and avoid possible biases.

A medicine based clinical practice and the rational application of these novel techniques (doing the essential exhaustive screening in order to select the best candidates to gain clinical benefit) will balance the performing of these promising procedures with more or less demonstrated results and the enormous commercial pressure that these devices development and researching suffer. We cannot forget the international economic situation that we are witnessing at this moment and we must show ourselves with clinical common sense enough to ensure maximum efficiency. If this is not guaranteed, exaggerated expenses and bad clinical results might lead to fail in the introduction of promising innovations before they are really tested.

As transcatheter aortic valve implantation techniques are spreading, newer indications for their use are extending with excellent initial results. That is the case of biological aortic prosthesis degeneration after conventional cardiac surgery. The anchoring of the transcatheter valve over the degenerated prosthesis seems to be quite safe and facilitate the treatment of patients that cannot undergo a surgical reintervention. We must wait until large series results to be reported before extract conclusions, but this is an obvious new field for the application of TAVI that can give response to an emerging problem as the population of developed countries keeps on aging.

3.7 Mid and long term follow-up results

There are relatively few data about mid and long-term follow-up results after transcatheter aortic valve implantation. The one-year survival after transfemoral implantation has reached 80% ore over in the most recent registries like SOURCE. It is interesting to remark the late publication in this sense of Webb et al where the majority of deaths that appear after 30 days are demonstrated to be non-cardiac related. This fact underlines again the main importance of making a proper patient selection in order to achieve good long-term results. Canadian multicentre experience (Rodés-Cadau J et al., 2010), that included transfemoral and transapical access, demonstrated that the presence of extra-cardiac comorbidities as renal failure or chronic obstructive pulmonary disease were two of the most importantly late mortality related factors. Finally, with the available data until date, no structural damage has been found yet in the mid-term follow up.

Recent long-term results of a single centre have been reported with the transfemoral CoreValve system in 450 patients. Pre-procedure logistic EuroSCORE was over 20% in >90% of the cohort. Early in-hospital mortality has been decreasing during last two years until stabilization in 6%. Other in-hospital complications have decreased as well with the exemption of pacemaker requirements that stabilizes in 39%. Stroke appeared in 1,6% of the patients. One-year survival was 60% with the 25F device, 79% with the 21F and 84% with the 18F, remarking the critical importance that the design improvement holds.

Transapical procedures have been related to one-year survival rates <80%, even in recent registries as SOURCE, probably due to higher risk basal characteristics of patients selected for this approach. Lichtenstein et al reported their initial experience in seven severe aortic stenosis patients that presented bad vascular access and severe comorbidities (Lichtenstein et al., 2006). Valve was implanted through a minimal thoracic incision and apex puncture without cardiopulmonary by-pass. There was no early mortality or valve dysfunction in this report. One year later, Walther et al reported their initial experience in a 30 patients cohort. Valve implantation was successfully implanted in 29 and one patient required cardiac surgery conversion with median sternotomy. After these reports, the possibility for an alternative access route when lack of vascular access is present was demonstrated. The same late author reported the experience of 4 centres that treated 59 patients with a mean EuroSCORE of 24±14% intended for Edwards-Sapien transcatheter heart valve implantation. Procedure was performed successfully in 53 patients when 4 patients required sternotomy and standard surgery conversion. Early in-hospital mortality was 13,6% and no prosthesis dysfunction was observed. (Walther T et al 2007)

Out of Europe, four American centres also reported their initial experience with the first 40 Edwards-Sapien implantation tries. The valve was successfully implanted in 35 patients. 30-days mortality was 17,5% and in a 143 days follow-up 6 more patients died, so Kaplan-Meier curves showed survival rates of 81,8±6,2% at one month, and 71,7±7,7% at 3 months.

The PARTNER EU registry included 69 severe aortic stenosis patients with serious comorbidities, high-risk surgical profile (mean logistic EuroSCORE 33,8±14,7%) and poor vascular access. Technical device implantation success was achieved in 91%. 30-days mortality was 18,8%; stroke 2,9%, conversion to standard surgery 2,9% and permanent pacemaker 4,4%. On-year survival was 50% and an important improvement in functional class was recognized for the majority of patients.

The largest cohort of transapical Edwards-Sapien implantation is the one in the SOURCE registry, with 575 patients. Mean logistic EuroSCORE was 29,2% and primary procedure success was reached in 92,8%. Conversion to standard surgery was reported in 3,5%, severe aortic regurgitation in 5,9an valve malaposition in 1,4%. 30-days mortality was 10,3%, stroke 2,9% and permanent pacemaker implantation 7,3%.

Medical industry has found in TAVI an open door for alternative treatment demands, so many companies are promoting research and developing of newer devices at this moment. Sadra Lotus, Direct Flow, Sorin Perceval, 3F Endurance Valve, LPI Repositionable, Lutter Valve, Heart Leaflet Technologies, Aortech and Artx valves may serve as an example.

Summarizing, we are now witnessing the beginning of a new era in the development of therapies for patients affected of aortic stenosis. The rigorous selection of patients and the rigorous obtaining of clinical data from trials and registries will determine the permanence and rising of this highly promising short of therapies.

4. Sutureless biological aortic valve surgical replacement

Clinical short and long term results of conventional aortic valve replacement have been clearly established along the last decades. At this moment, medical industry is developing a new short of biological aortic valve prosthesis that, despite the standard cardiopulmonary by-pass and aortic clamping need, they hold the advantage of a sutureless implantation system that leads to a faster surgery with less on-pump time with the evident benefits in terms of surgical risks. Interesting alternative application of sutureless valves is the redo surgery (re-interventions after prosthesis dysfunction). In this short of surgery, as it is always complex and risky, reducing aortic clamping time is essential, so these sutereless valves may offer an inestimable help by accelerating the valve insertion process. In case of biological dysfunctional prosthesis, sutereless valves allow a valve-in-valve implantation without the extraction of the previous dysfunctional valve. This procedure is performed by deployment of the sutureless valve within the pre-implanted valve stent-annulus, avoiding this way the risks involved in prosthesis removal (aortic root and annulus manipulation and prolonging clamping time).

This kind of prosthesis generate very low hemodynamic gradient because they are constructed over a low profile metallic stent, with a similar structure to transcatheter-deployable devices. This advantage improves valve hemodynamics and may contribute to ventricular mass regression.

The commercial bid of this group of prosthesis is based on its capacity to reduce the aggression of standard surgery, favouring the realization of progressively less invasive surgical techniques (ministernotomy, minithoracotomy, robotic surgery…) and the adding value of its contribution on the researching and development of future transcatheter devices.

Sorin´s Perceval and 3F´s Enable are the more promising models at this moment. The companies involved in the production of this prosthesis are those who may point the aim of this technique: development of newer transcatheter devices or really improve standard surgery results.(Shrestha M et al., 2009, Aymard T et al., 2010)

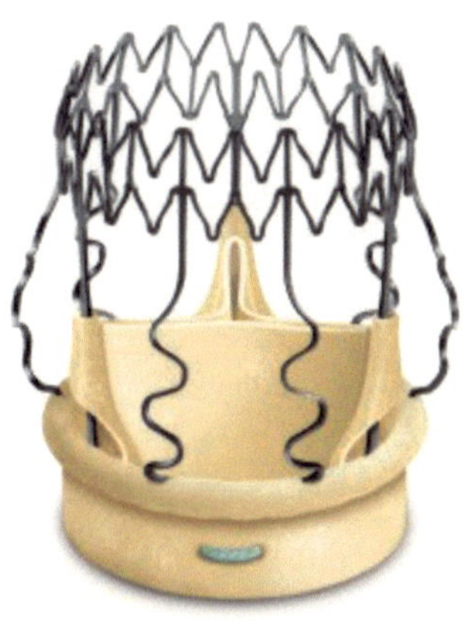

Perceval Sorin Valve

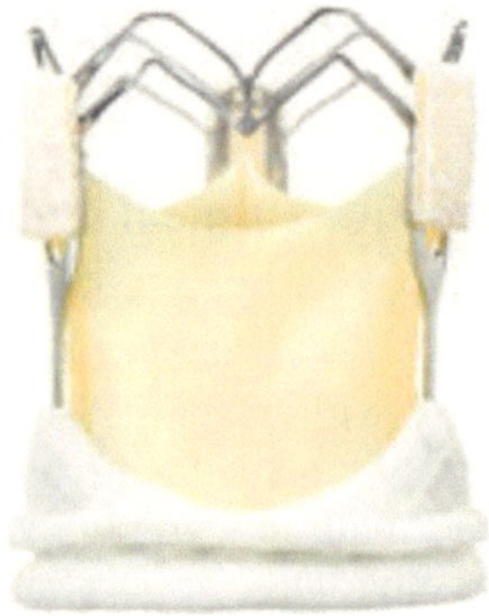

Enable 3F Valve

5. Apicoaortic conduits

Surgical aortic valve replacement by median thoracotomy under cardiopulmonary bypass is, as mentioned above, the standard therapy for severe aortic stenosis that has proven superiority to conservative pharmacological therapy. Many times, however, this treatment cannot be performed because of different technical, anatomic or clinical problems that the patient may present, as it could be porcelain aorta or tiny aortic annulus. Aortic valve conduits, also known as apicoaortic conduits, are a short of devices designed in the sixties to give an alternative in these situations. Apicoaortic conduits connect the left ventricle apex with the descending thoracic aorta, relieving the intraventricular pressure by allowing the blood flow to find a way out of the heart without fighting against the aortic valve resistance. Because the operation was technically difficult, it had fallen into disuse, but, with the introduction of technically easier and less invasive procedures performed by minithoracotomy, this alternative offers clear advantages over standard valve replacement (avoidance of sternotomy, cardiopulmonary bypass, cardioplegic cardiac arrest, native valve debridement, conduction system injury, aortic cannulation, and aortic cross-clamping) and arises as another option in addition to transcatheter aortic valve implantation as alternative therapy for high risk patients. This technique offers the possibility to choose from a big variety of valve models and sizes, it

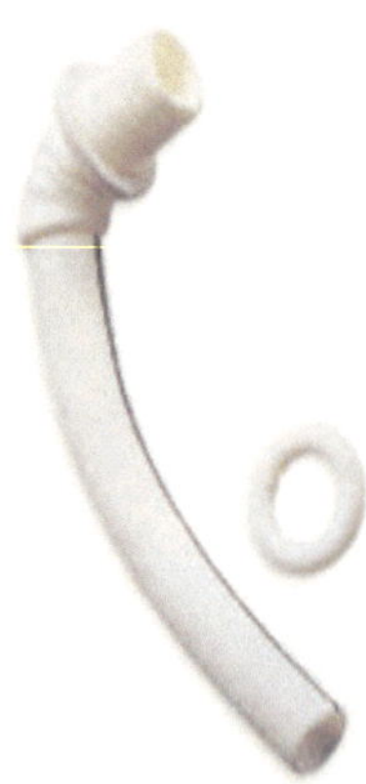

Aorto-apical conduit Medtronic Hancock

has proven long-term efficacy and durability, involves lower peri-procedural stroke risk and has no incremented AV block or paravalvular leak risks. As disadvantage, it commonly requires cardiopulmonary bypass pump, though some off-pump cases have been reported (Vassiliades TA Jr et al 2003; Hirota M et al; Chahine JH et al., 2009)

6. Conclusions

As the developed countries population continues its progressive aging, number of patients grows as the majority of cases, with the subsequent increase in co-morbidities and risk profile worsening. In the other hand, technical improvements and innovation in newer devices design and performance make these alternatives more and more attractive. In this scenario, the data reported by big clinical trials as PARTNER may result in a deep revolution in degenerative aortic stenosis management, where minimal invasive procedures arise as the procedures of choice for this high-risk population. We must wait until definitive publications in this way before introducing any change in the clinical practice guidelines, but at this moment we can be quite confident about the fact these novel techniques "are here to stay"

7. References

Andersen HR, Knudsen LL, Hasenkam JM. Transluminal implantation of artificial heart valves. Description of a new expandable aortic valve and initial results with implantation by catheter technique in closed chest pigs. Eur Heart J. 1992 May;13 (5):704–708.

Alexander KP, Anstrom KJ, Muhlbaier LH, Grosswald RD, Smith PK, Jones RH, et al. Outcomes of cardiac surgery in patients >80 years; results from the National Cardiovascular Network. J Am Coll Cardiol. 2000 Mar; 35 (3):731-8.

Aregger F, Wenaweser P, Hellige GJ, Kadner A, Carrel T, Windecker S, et al. Risk of acute kidney injury in patients with severe aortic valve stenosis undergoing transcatheter valve replacement. Nephrol Dial Transplant. 2009 Jul;24 (7):2175-9.

Aymard T, Kadner A, Walpoth N, Göber V, Englberger L, Stalder M, Eckstein F, Zobrist C, Carrel T. Clinical experience with the second-generation 3f Enable sutureless aortic valve prosthesis. J Thorac Cardiovasc Surg. 2010 Aug;140(2):313-6

Bagur R, Webb JG, Nietlispach F, Dumont E, De Larochellière R, Doyle D, et al. Acute kidney injury following transcatheter aortic valve implantation: predictive factors, prognostic value, and comparison with surgical aortic valve replacement. Eur Heart J. 2010 Apr;31(7):865-74.

Bagur R, Dumont E, Doyle D, Larose E, Lemieux J, Bergeron S, et al. Coronary ostia stenosis following transcatheter aortic valve implantation. JACC Cardiovasc Interv. 2010 Feb; 3:253-5.

Bonhoeffer P, Boudjemline Y, Saliba Z, Merckz J, Yacine A, Bonnet D, et al. Percutaneous replacement of pulmonary valve in a right ventricle to pulmonary-artery prosthetic conduit with valve dysfunction. Lancet. 2000 Oct 21;356:1403-5.

Buellesfeld L, Wenaweser P, Gerckens U, Mueller R, Sauren B, Latsios G, et al. Transcatheter aortic valve implantation: predictors of procedural success—the Siegburg-Bern experience. Eur Heart J. 2010 Apr;31(8):984-91.

Chahine JH, El-Rassi I, Jebara V. Apico-aortic valved conduit as an alternative for aortic valve re-replacement in severe prosthesis-patient mismatch. Interact Cardiovasc Thorac Surg. 2009 Oct;9(4):680-2.

Charlson E, Legedza ATR, Hamel MB. Decision-making and outcomes in severe symptomatic aortic stenosis. J Heart Valve Dis. 2006 May;15 (3):312–321.

Cribier A, Eltchaninoff H, Bash A, Borenstein N, Tron C, Bauer F, Derumeaux G, Anselme F, Laborde F, Leon MB. Percutaneous transcatheter implantation of an aortic valve prosthesis for calcific aortic stenosis: first human case description. Circulation. 2002 Dec 10;106:3006–3008.

Cribier A, Eltchaninoff H, Tron C, Bauer F, Agatiello C, Nercolini D, et al. Treatment of calcific aortic stenosis with the percutaneous heart valve. Mid-term follow-up from the initial feasibility studies: the French experience. J Am Coll Cardiol. 2006 Mar 21;47:1214-23.

Delgado V, Ng AC, Shanks M, van der Kley F, Schuijf JD, van de Veire NR, Kroft L, de Roos A, Schalij MJ, Bax JJ. Transcatheter aortic valve implantation: role of multimodality cardiac imaging. Expert Rev Cardiovasc Ther. 2010 Jan;8(1):113-23.

Dumont E, Lemieux J, Doyle D, Rodés-Cabau J. Feasibility of transapical aortic valve implantation fully guided by transesophageal echocardiography. J Thorac Cardiovasc Surg. 2009 Oct ;138:1022-4.

Grube E, Buellesfeld L, Mueller R, Sauren B, Zickmann B, Nair D, et al. Progress and current status of percutaneous aortic valve replacement results of three device generations of the CoreValve Revalving system. Circ Cardiovasc Interv. 2008 Dec;1:167-75.

Grube E, Laborde JC, Zickmann B, Gerckens U, Felderhoff T, Sauren B, et al. First report on a human percutaneous transluminal implantation of a self-expanding valve prosthesis for interventional treatment of aortic valve stenosis. Catheter Cardiovasc Interv. 2005 Dec;66:465-9.

Himbert D, Descoutures F, Al-Attar N, Iung B, Ducrocq G, Détaint D, et al. Results of transfemoral or transapical aortic valve implantation following a uniform assessment in high-risk patients with aortic stenosis. J Am Coll Cardiol. 2009 Jul 21;54:303-11.

Hirota M, Oi M, Omoto T, Tedoriya T. Apico-aortic conduit for aortic stenosis with a porcelain aorta; technical modification for apical outflow. Interact Cardiovasc Thorac Surg. 2009 Oct;9(4):703-5.

Iung B, Baron G, Butchart EG, Delahaye F, Gohlke-Barwolf C, Levang OW, Tornos P, Vanoverschelde JL, Vermeer F, Boersma E, Ravaud P, Vahanian A. A prospective survey of patients with valvular heart disease in Europe: the Euro Heart Survey on Valvular Heart Disease. Eur Heart J.2003 Jul; 24 (13):1231–1243.

Jilaihawi H, Chin D, Vasa-Nicotera M, Jeilam M, Spyt T, Ng GA, et al. Predictors for permanent pacemaker requirement after transcatheter aortic valve implantation with the CoreValve bioprosthesis. Am Heart J. 2009 Apr;157:860-6.

Kapadia SR, Svensson L, Tuzcu M. Successful percutaneous management of left main trunk occlusion during percutaneous aortic valve replacement. Catheter Cardiovasc Intervent. 2009 Jun 1;73:966-72

Kvidal P, Bergströn R, Hórte LG, Stahle E. Observed and relative survival after aortic valve replacement. J Am Coll Cardiol. 2000 Mar; 35 (3):747-56.

Kempfert J, Falk V, Schuler G, Linke A, Merk D, Mohr FW, Walther T. Dyna-CT during minimally invasive off-pump transapical aortic valve implantation. Ann Thorac Surg. 2009 Dec;88(6):2041.

Kodali SK, O'Neill WW, Moses JW, Williams M, Smith CR, Tuzcu M, Svensson LG, Kapadia S, Hanzel G, Kirtane AJ, Leon MB. Early and Late (One Year) Outcomes Following Transcatheter Aortic Valve Implantation in Patients With Severe Aortic Stenosis (from the United States REVIVAL Trial). Am J Cardiol. 2011 Apr 1;107(7):1058-64.

Ng AC, Delgado V, van der Kley F, Shanks M, van de Veire NR, Bertini M, Nucifora G, van Bommel RJ, Tops LF, de Weger A, Tavilla G, de Roos A, Kroft LJ, Leung DY, Schuijf J, Schalij MJ, Bax JJ. Comparison of aortic root dimensions and geometries before and after transcatheter aortic valve implantation by 2- and 3-dimensional transesophageal echocardiography and multislice computed tomography. Circ Cardiovasc Imaging. 2010 Jan;3(1):94-102.

Leon MB, Smith CR, Mack M, Miller DC, Moses JW, Svensson LG, Tuzcu EM, Webb JG, Fontana GP, Makkar RR, Brown DL, Block PC, Guyton RA, Pichard AD, Bavaria JE, Herrmann HC, Douglas PS, Petersen JL, Akin JJ, Anderson WN, Wang D, Pocock S; PARTNER Trial Investigators. Transcatheter aortic-valve implantation for aortic stenosis in patients who cannot undergo surgery. N Engl J Med. 2010 Oct 21;363(17):1597-607.

Pai RG, Kapoor N, Bansal RC, Varadarajan P. Malignant natural history of asymptomatic severe aortic stenosis: benefit of aortic valve replacement. Ann Thorac Surg. 2006 Dec; 82 (6):2116–2122.

Piazza N, Onuma Y, Jesserun E, Kint PP, Maugenest AM, Anderson RH, et al. Early and persistent intraventricular conduction abnormalities and requirements for pacemaking after percutaneous replacement of the aortic valve. JACC Cardiovasc Interv. 2008 Jun;1:310-6.

Rodés-Cabau J, Dumont E, DelaRochellière R, Doyle D, Lemieux J, Bergeron S, et al. Feasibility and initial results of percutaneous aortic valve implantation including selection of the transfemoral or transapical approach in patients with severe aortic stenosis. Am J Cardiol. 2008 Nov;102 (9):1240-4.

Rodés-Cabau J, Webb JB, Anson C, Ye J, Dumont E, Feindel C, et al. Transcatheter aortic valve implantation for the treatment of severe symptomatic aortic stenosis in patients at very high or prohibitive surgical risk. Acute and late outcomes of the multicenter Canadian experience. J Am Coll Cardiol. 2010 Mar 16;55:1080-90.

Shrestha M, Folliguet T, Meuris B, Dibie A, Bara C, Herregods MC, Khaladj N, Hagl C, Flameng W, Laborde F, Haverich A. Sutureless Perceval S aortic valve replacement: a multicenter, prospective pilot trial. J Heart Valve Dis. 2009 Nov;18(6):698-702.

Thomas M, Schymik G, Walther T, Himbert D, Lefèvre T, Treede H, Eggebrecht H, Rubino P, Michev I, Lange R, Anderson WN, Wendler O. Thirty-day results of the SAPIEN aortic Bioprosthesis European Outcome (SOURCE) Registry: A European registry of transcatheter aortic valve implantation using the Edwards SAPIEN valve. Circulation. 2010 Jul 6;122(1):62-9.

Varadarajan P, Kapoor N, Bansal RC, Pai RG. Clinical profile and natural history of 453 nonsurgically managed patients with severe aortic stenosis. Ann Thorac Surg. 2006 Dec; 82 (6):2111–2115.

Vahanian A, Palacios IF. Percutaneous approaches to valvular disease. Circulation. 2004 April 6;109:1572-9.

Vahanian A, Baumgartner H, Bax J, Butchart E, Dion R, Filippatos G, Flachskampf F, Hall R, Iung B, Kasprzak J, Nataf P, Tornos P, Torracca L, Wenink A; Guidelines on the management of valvular heart disease: The Task Force on the Management of Valvular Heart Disease of the European Society of Cardiology. Task Force on the Management of Valvular Hearth Disease of the European Society of Cardiology; ESC Committee for Practice Guidelines. Eur Heart J. 2007 Jan;28(2):230-68.

Vahanian A, Alfieri O, Al-Attar N, Antunes M, Bax J, Cormier B, Cribier A, De Jaegere P, Fournial G, Kappetein AP, Kovac J, Ludgate S, Maisano F, Moat N, Mohr F, Nataf P, Piérard L, Pomar JL, Schofer J, Tornos P, Tuzcu M, van Hout B, Von Segesser LK, Walther T; Transcatheter valve implantation for patients with aortic stenosis: a position statement from the European Association of Cardio-Thoracic Surgery (EACTS) and the European Society of Cardiology (ESC), in collaboration with the European Association of Percutaneous Cardiovascular Interventions (EAPCI). European Association of Cardio-Thoracic Surgery; European Society of Cardiology; European Association of Percutaneous Cardiovascular Interventions. Eur Heart J. 2008 Jun;29(11):1463-70.

Vassiliades TA Jr. Off-pump apicoaortic conduit insertion for high-risk patients with aortic stenosis. Eur J Cardiothorac Surg. 2003 Feb;23(2):156-8.

Walther T, Simon P, Dewey T, Wimmer-Greinecker G, Falk V, Kasimir MT, et al. Transapical minimally invasive aortic valve implantation. Multicenter experience. Circulation. 2007 Sep 11;116:I240-5.

Webb JG, Chandavimol M, Thompson CR, Ricci DR, Carere RG, Munt BI, Buller CE, Pasupati S, Lichtenstein S. Percutaneous aortic valve implantation retrograde from the femoral artery. Circulation.2006 Feb 14;113:842–850.

Webb JG, Pasupati S, Humphries K, Thompson C, Altwegg L, Moss R, Sinhal A, Carere RG, Munt B, Ricci D, Ye J, Cheung A, Lichtenstein SV. Percutaneous transarterial aortic valve replacement in selected high-risk patients with aortic stenosis. Circulation. 2007 Aug 14;116:755–763.

Wendler O, Walther T, Nataf P, Rubino P, Schroefel H, Thielmann M, Treede H, Thomas M. Trans-apical aortic valve implantation: univariate and multivariate analyses of the early results from the SOURCE registry. Eur J Cardiothorac Surg. 2010 Aug;38(2):119-27.

Wood D, Tops LF, Mayo JR, Pasupati S, Schalij MJ, Humphries K, et al. Role of multislice computed tomography in transcatheter aortic valve replacement. Am J Cardiol. 2009 May 1;103:1295-301.